Exercise Leadership in Cardiac Rehabilitation

An

Exercise Leadership in Cardiac Rehabilitation

An evidence-based approach

Edited by Morag K. Thow Dip PE, BSc, PhD, MCSP
Lecturer in Physiotherapy, Glasgow Caledonian University
Glasgow, UK

John Wiley & Sons, Ltd

Telephone (+44) 1243 779777

Email (for orders and customer service enquiries): cs-books@wiley.co.uk
Visit our Home Page on www.wiley.com

Reprinted November 2006

Other Wiley Editorial Offices

John Wiley & Sons Inc., 111 River Street, Hoboken, NJ 07030, USA

Jossey-Bass, 989 Market Street, San Francisco, CA 94103-1741, USA

Wiley-VCH Verlag GmbH, Boschstr. 12, D-69469 Weinheim, Germany

John Wiley & Sons Australia Ltd, 42 McDougall Street, Milton, Queensland 4064, Australia

John Wiley & Sons (Asia) Pte Ltd, 2 Clementi Loop #02-01, Jin Xing Distripark, Singapore 129809

John Wiley & Sons Canada Ltd, 22 Worcester Road, Etobicoke, Ontario, Canada M9W 1L1

Wiley also publishes its books in a variety of electronic formats. Some content that appears in print may not be available in electronic books.

Library of Congress Cataloging-in-Publication Data
Exercise leadership in Cardiac Rehabilitation: An evidence based approach / [edited by] Morag K Thow.
   p. ; cm.
  Includes bibliographical references and index.
  ISBN 0-470-01971-9 (pbk.)
  1. Heart – Diseases – Patients – Rehabilitation. 2. Evidence-based medicine.
  [DNLM: 1. Heart Diseases – rehabilitation. 2. Evidence-Based Medicine.
  3. Exercise Therapy – methods. WG 166 C2638 2006] I. Thow, Morag K. II. Title.
  RC681.C1798 2006
  616.1′203 – dc22

                                                2005025382

British Library Cataloguing in Publication Data

A catalogue record for this book is available from the British Library

ISBN-13 978-0-470-01971-9 (PB)

Typeset by SNP Best-set Typesetter Ltd., Hong Kong
Printed and bound in Great Britain by TJ International Ltd, Padstow, Cornwall
This book is printed on acid-free paper responsibly manufactured from sustainable forestry in which at least two trees are planted for each one used for paper production.

I would like to dedicate this book to Alex and Sylvia Johnston who were our first cardiac rehabilitation participants at Gartnavel General Hospital, Glasgow. Also to all the other cardiac rehabilitation participants and partners at Jordanhill Heartbeats who have given me as much as I hope I have given them.

Contents

Contributors ix

Foreword xi

Preface xiii

Acknowledgements xv

1 Cardiac Rehabilitation Overview 1
  Christine Proudfoot

2 Risk Stratification and Health Screening for Exercise
  in Cardiac Rehabilitation 19
  Ann Ross and Mhairi Campbell

3 Exercise Physiology and Monitoring of Exercise in Cardiac
  Rehabilitation 47
  John Buckley

4 Exercise Prescription in Cardiac Rehabilitation 97
  Hilary Dingwall, Kim Ferrier and Joanne Semple

5 Class Design and Use of Music in Cardiac Rehabilitation 133
  Linda Harley and Gillian Armstrong

6 Leadership, Exercise Class Management and Safety in Cardiac
  Rehabilitation 161
  Fiona Lough

7 Teaching Skills for Cardiac Rehabilitation Exercise Classes 183
  Morag K. Thow

8 Maintaining Physical Activity in Cardiac Rehabilitation 195
  Adrienne Hughes and Nanette Mutrie

Appendix A – Glossary 219

Index 223

Contributors

Gillian Armstrong BSc MCSP
Senior Physiotherapist, Cardiac Rehabilitation, Glasgow Royal Infirmary, University NHS Glasgow, 16 Alexandra Parade, Glasgow, G31 2ER.

John Buckley BPE MSc PhD
Lecturer in Exercise Science, School of Health and Rehabilitation, Keele University, Staffordshire, ST5 5BG.

Mhairi Campbell, BSc MCSP
Cardiac Rehabilitation Co-ordinator, Health at Heart Centre, Royal Alexandra Hospital, NHS Paisley, Corsebar Road, Paisley, PA2 9PN.

Hilary Dingwall BSc MCSP
Superintendent Physiotherapist, Cardiac Rehabilitation, Victoria Infirmary University NHS Glasgow, Langside, Glasgow, G42 9TY.

Kim Ferrier BSc MCSP
Senior Physiotherapist, Cardiac Rehabilitation, Glasgow Royal Infirmary, University NHS Glasgow, 16 Alexandra Parade, Glasgow, G31 2ER.

Linda Harley RGN
Cardiac Specialist Nurse, Vale of Leven District Hospital NHS, Main Street, Alexandria, G83 OUA.

Adrienne Hughes PhD
Research Fellow, University Department, Human Nutrition, Yorkhill Hospital NHS Glasgow, G3 8SJ.

Fiona Lough MPhil MCSP
Superintendent Physiotherapist, Cardiac Rehabilitation, University College London NHS, London, WC1E 6AU.

Nanette Mutrie PhD FBASES
Professor, Department of Sport, Culture and the Arts, Strathclyde University, PESO Building, Glasgow, G13 1PP.

Christine Proudfoot MSc MCSP
Senior Physiotherapist, Cardiac Rehabilitation, Hairmyres Hospital NHS, East Kilbride, G4 8RG.

Ann Ross MPhil MCSP
Superintendent Physiotherapist, Western Infirmary University NHS, Glasgow, Dumbarton Road, Glasgow, G11 6NT.

Joanne Semple BSc MCSP
Senior Physiotherapist, Cardiac Rehabilitation, Southern General NHS Glasgow.

Morag K. Thow PhD MCSP
Lecturer in Physiotherapy, Glasgow Caledonian University, Cowcaddens Road, Glasgow G4 OBA.

Foreword

EXERCISE LEADERSHIP IN CARDIAC REHABILITATION

The benefits of cardiac rehabilitation are now well established in a wide range of patients with cardiac disease. A cardiac rehabilitation programme is a vehicle for the delivery of holistic secondary prevention and could be considered as one method of chronic disease management. This includes risk factor modification, prescription of appropriate medication and health behaviour change. It therefore consists of a series of evidenced based interventions designed to optimise these outcome for patients. Although several meta analysis have shown mortality benefits from exercise based cardiac rehabilitation programmes, the evaluation of modern programmes should focus on the outcomes described above and hospital re-admission. Cardiac rehabilitation programmes should be tailored to the individual needs of the patient and extended to the broader group of cardiac patients a step change in their condition. Programmes must deliver evidence based practise and adhere to national guidelines. However research and development should be encouraged and supported. Audit of cardiac rehabilitation programmes, using nationally agreed datasets is essential to measure outcomes, inform programme development and secure resources.

This book entitled Exercise Leadership in Cardiac Rehabilitation is a comprehensive account of the exercise component of health behaviour change within cardiac rehabilitation. It is written by clinicians for clinicians and contains a practical guide to exercise prescription. The book will be invaluable to clinicians involved in cardiac rehabilitation and will facilitate programme development.

By Dr Paul.D.MacIntyre
Consultant Cardiologist
RAH

Preface

Cardiac rehabilitation (CR) is now established as part of cardiac care in the UK, and is embedded in many government policies and national guidelines, with structured exercise as a key element. Over the last ten years there has been a radical shift in the provision of exercise-based CR in the UK. Government recommendations and national guidelines encompass the traditional post myocardial infarction (MI) and revascularisation groups, but also the older patient and the more complex cardiac groups, including those with heart failure and angina. The diversity of CR patients puts new and demanding challenges on the exercise leader of CR.

In 20 years of research and development of CR programmes in the UK I have become aware that there is no definitive book that provides physiotherapists and exercise professionals with a comprehensive resource on the exercise components and skills of constructing and teaching CR exercise. The objective of this text is to address the scope of knowledge and skills required of exercise specialists developing, delivering and teaching exercise-based CR programmes. The book is structured on an evidence-based theoretical framework, but also provides practical advice and suggestions based on the clinical experience of the contributing authors, thus providing physiotherapists and exercise professionals with a comprehensive practical text that can be used to plan, develop and deliver exercise-based CR in all phase of CR.

The book starts with a chapter which overviews the historical and contemporary context of CR, including a brief overview of the potential benefits of exercise in the CR patients. This is followed by Chapter 2 on medical aspects and risk stratification for the exercise component for the different groups of CR patients. This leads to Chapter 3 which addresses exercise physiology and monitoring issues. Chapter 4 focuses on exercise prescription and class structures applicable to the spectrum of patients included in exercise-based CR. Chapter 5 deals with design of classes and use of music. Chapter 6 deals with the organisational and management role of the exercise specialist. This is followed by a key chapter addressing the skills of group exercise teaching, which are neglected in other publications on CR. The final chapter is dedicated to adult exercise behaviour and exercise consultation, required to help patients and families adopt and sustain exercise as part of their health behaviour.

Each section, where appropriate, is evidence-based and fully referenced. Furthermore, where appropriate, useful templates and material are provided so that readers can easily transfer the material into their programmes. The book is designed and constructed to be used and read as a whole, but each section and/or chapter can stand alone. Furthermore, there are chapters within the text that are applicable to and can be transferred to other exercise teaching contexts for example, pulmonary rehabilitation (PR).

The physiotherapist and exercise specialist are in a key position within CR to provide exercise, advice and support. This book will help them meet the challenges of the range of cardiac patients in their exercise classes and will help them 'make a difference' in meeting the challenges of exercise leadership in CR.

Acknowledgements

I would like to acknowledge all the contributing authors who have been generous with their time, knowledge and experience. I would also like to thank Dr Rowena Murray for her practical support and her encouragement to finish this book. Finally, I would like to thank and acknowledge Danny Rafferty, Gordon Morland, Gayle Mackie, John McGuinness, Lorna Ross and John Reid for their technical and practical help over the years.

Chapter 1

Cardiac Rehabilitation Overview

Christine Proudfoot

Chapter outline

Cardiac rehabilitation (CR) is now established as part of cardiac care in the UK and is embedded in many government policies and national guidelines, with structured exercise as a key element. This chapter reviews the incidence and pattern of coronary heart disease presentation in the UK. In addition, the spectrum of patient groups included in CR is reviewed. The chapter defines the content of contemporary CR, reviews the evidence base for exercise in comprehensive CR and sets the scene for the chapters that follow.

DEFINITION OF CARDIAC REHABILITATION

There are many aspects to the management of coronary heart disease (CHD), including pharmacological treatment, cardiac investigations, secondary prevention and revascularisation. Secondary prevention consists of a number of activities or measures that may be taken by patients with established disease, in order to reduce their risk of a further event (Lockhart, *et al.*, 2000). Cardiac rehabilitation (CR) is acknowledged not only as integral in the management of patients with CHD, but also as the primary vehicle in delivering secondary prevention. Many definitions of CR exist, for example the World Health Organisation classifies CR as 'The sum of activities required to influence favourably the underlying cause of the disease, as well as to ensure the patient the best possible physical, mental and social conditions, so that they may, by their own efforts, preserve or resume when lost, as normal a place as possible in the life of the community' (World Health Organisation, 1993).

Exercise Leadership in Cardiac Rehabilitation. An Evidence-Based Approach. Edited by Morag Thow.
Copyright 2006 by John Wiley & Sons Ltd. ISBN 0-470-01971-9

More recently CR has been redefined by the Scottish Intercollegiate Guidelines Network, subsequently adopted by the British Association for Cardiac Rehabilitation (BACR) as the UK guideline, as follows: 'Cardiac rehabilitation is the process by which patients with cardiac disease, in partnership with a multidisciplinary team of health professionals, are encouraged and supported to achieve and maintain optimal physical and psychosocial health' (SIGN, 2002). This is perhaps a more succinct definition, which encompasses all the key elements of CR, such as partnership, support, and the aim of optimising and maintaining the individual's health. Furthermore, the SIGN (2002) guideline acknowledges the key role that exercise plays in contemporary CR.

CORONARY HEART DISEASE

Over the last ten years the pattern of CHD mortality and morbidity has changed with premature death rates reduced but more survivors of myocardial infarction (MI) (BHF, 2003, 2004).

CHD mortality

In 2002, there were approximately 40 000 premature deaths from CHD in the UK (BHF, 2004). This rate is amongst the highest in the world. Within the UK there are also regional differences with death rates highest in Scotland and the North of England and lowest in the South of England (BHF, 2004). There is some positive evidence that the death rates from CHD have been falling in the UK in the last ten years. For example, in adults under 65 years, the rate has fallen by 44% (BHF, 2004). This is not as fast as some other countries, with Australia and Norway both showing a decreasing death rate for men aged 35–74 of 47% (BHF, 2004). Although there is an overall improvement in the statistics for the UK, there is no room for complacency.

Fifty-eight per cent of the reduction in mortality over the past 20 years in the UK can be explained by the reduction of major risk factors, principally smoking (BHF, 2004). Other early pharmacological interventions and secondary prevention account for the remaining reduction of the mortality decline. Secondary prevention and the contribution of CR can also be associated with reduction on mortality (Jolliffe, *et al.*, 2004; Taylor, *et al.*, 2004; Leon, *et al.*, 2005).

CHD morbidity

Studies have shown that the incidence rate of MI is between 2 and 2.5 times the mortality rate, and using data from 2002 it is estimated that in all ages, a total of 268 000 people (147 000 men and 121 000 women) in the UK had an MI in 2002 (BHF, 2004). Prevalence of MI increases with age and is higher in men than in women; estimates show that there are about 838 000 men and 394 000 women living in the UK, who have had an MI (BHF, 2004). The prevalence of MI is disproportionately higher in Scotland: 43 per 1000 men, compared with 39 in Wales and 34 in England (Wanless, 2001; SIGN, 2002). In addition, there is an increasing number of MI and CHD subjects with chronic heart failure (HF), approximately 662 000 in the UK (BHF, 2004).

In addition, the BHF (BHF, 2004) estimate 178 000 new cases of angina in all men living in the UK and about 159 500 in women, totalling 337 500. As can be seen from the trends in the increase in morbidity, there is more need for structured secondary prevention. As CR is recognised as the prime vehicle for delivery of secondary prevention (SIGN, 2002), there will be a corresponding increase in comprehensive, patient-centred CR.

PATIENT GROUPS IN CARDIAC REHABILITATION

Traditionally post-MI and revascularisation patients were referred for CR (SIGN, 2002). There are now many more groups included in exercise-based CR. In addition, definition of MI has changed with the introduction of troponin blood tests.

Acute coronary syndromes

Acute coronary syndromes include unstable angina, non-ST-segment elevation MI (NSTE MI) and ST-segment elevation MI (STE MI) (Santiago and Tadros, 2002). It is acknowledged that with revised definition of myocardial infarction, diagnosed by cardiac troponin estimation, there will be a resultant increase in the reporting of myocardial infarction, with increased workloads for the services involved (Dalal, *et al.*, 2004). In the Cochrane systematic review by Jolliffe, *et al.* (2004) the reviewers concluded that exercise-based CR is effective in reducing cardiac deaths and has many positive health-related outcomes for post-MI and CHD groups.

Post-revascularisation

Comprehensive CR is recommended for patients who have undergone revascularisation that includes coronary artery bypass grafting and percutaneous intervention (angioplasty and stenting) (SIGN, 2002). There can be a misconception by patients that the revascularisation procedure has eradicated the underlying CHD process. It is important that this group of patients continues to address their CHD risk factors. Exercise-based CR has considerable impact on physiological and psychosocial cardiac risk factors post-revascularisation (Ross, *et al.*, 2000; Stewart, *et al.*, 2003).

Stable angina

There have been few studies on exercise and this group of patients compared to other cardiac groups. One of the first studies to investigate exercise in angina patients was by Todd, *et al.* (1991). They found that habitual exercise had an anti-anginal effect, with the subjects experiencing up to 34% reduction in ischaemia. The authors hypothesised that exercise training enhanced myocardial collateral function. Kligfield, *et al.* (2003) further suggested that sustained habitual exercise in this patient group enhances the parasympathetic tone of the heart. A review of literature by the Scottish Intercollegiate Guideline Network (SIGN, 2002) examining CR and patients with stable angina found that this patient group should be considered for CR if they have limiting symptoms. Angina patients appropriate for exercise-based CR may be those who are not suitable for revascularisation and/or have an anginal threshold of 4 METs or more (ACSM, 2000). The aim of exercise is to raise the ischaemic threshold and thus allow patients to exercise more before their angina occurs. In addition, efficent use of anti-anginal medication can help this group to carry out more exercise (Durstine and Moore, 2003).

Chronic heart failure

There are increasing numbers of patients presenting with heart failure and being referred to CR. Because of the negative effects on quality of life for these patients due to dyspnoea on exertion and fatigue and the generally poor prognosis, the interest in optimising the management of this patient group is increasing. The review of controlled trials of physical training in chronic heart failure by the European Heart Failure Group (1998) concluded that there are positive effects of physical rehabilitation in stable heart failure patients on function and quality of life. A further systematic review of evidence by Lloyd-Williams, *et al.* (2002) found that short-term physical exercise training in selected subgroups of patients with chronic heart failure has physiological benefits and positive effects on quality of life. These findings are confirmed, with a collaborative meta-analysis, by ExTraMATCH (2004), providing evidence of an overall reduction in mortality for HF groups. The largest improvements in exercise capacity and quality of life are found in those patients with mild to moderate HF (Rees, *et al.*, 2004).

Cardiac transplantation

This is likely to be a small group of patients and the research examining cardiac transplantation and cardiac rehabilitation is not extensive. In the UK only the SIGN (2002) guidelines make specific mention of this patient group. An American study by Shephard (1998) suggested that there is a need for exercise-centred cardiac rehabilitation to optimise functional gains and counter major complications, such as hypertension, accelerated atherosclerosis and osteoporosis. The detrimental effects of muscle weakness are responsible for a substantial part of the initial functional disturbance, and rehabilitation programmes should include resistance and weight-bearing activities as well as aerobic exercise. Kobashigawa, *et al.* (1999) found that when initiated early after cardiac transplantation, exercise training increased capacity for physical work in transplant patients.

Valve surgery

This patient group includes all types of valve surgery. The typical patient in this group will be post-aortic or mitral valve replacement. The exercise part of cardiac rehabilitation plays a role in reversing the symptoms associated with deconditioning. A review by Stewart, *et al.* (2003) examining valve surgery and cardiac rehabilitation found that supervised exercise training in comprehensive CR was effective in increasing functional capacity and favourably modifying disease-related risk factors, decreasing symptoms and improving quality of life for valve patients. Although studies have been limited due to small sample size and lack of control groups, there is increasing evidence of the benefits of exercise-based CR for these patients.

Congenital heart disease

The patient group includes children and young people. Exercise and physical activity levels are dependent on the differing types of congenital heart disease. There may be barriers to exercise in this group, such as current symptoms, lack of interest in exercise and health fears (Swan and Hillis, 2000). A review by Brugemann, *et al.* (2004) found that patients with congenital heart disease should be included in multidisciplinary CR. In addition, physical training was found to be safe. A pre-training exercise test is required to determine specific and appropriate physical workload. Furthermore, education, psycho-social support and coping strategies to help reduce anxiety are essential parts of CR for this patient group. Paediatric specialists have advocated exercise-training programmes for children with congenital heart disease. A review of literature by Imms (2004) suggests that CR programmes for children should also promote occupational performance activity and integrate exercise into self-care and leisure activity.

Implanted cardioverter defibrillators

Though not all CR guidelines specifically suggest provision of cardiac rehabilitation for patients following insertion of an implanted cardioverter defibrillator, most of this patient group will have CHD in conjunction with their arrhythmic tendency. The United Kingdom-based National Institute for

Clinical Excellence (NICE) recommends a rehabilitative approach to after-care, which includes psychological preparation for living with an implanted cardioverter defibrillator (NICE, 2000). For most cardiac rehabilitation programmes, the numbers of patients seen with an implanted cardioverter defibrillator are likely to be small. Nevertheless, it is important that these patients receive appropriate CR. It has been acknowledged that there should be larger multi-centred studies on this group (NICE, 2000). There is some evidence that comprehensive CR is safe for patients with implanted cardioverter defibrillators and can improve exercising ability and lower levels of psychological distress (Fitchet, *et al.*, 2003; Vanhees, *et al.*, 2004).

Under-represented groups

Special consideration should be made for the elderly, women and minority ethnic groups to ensure that their particular needs are met. These groups tend to be under-represented in CR, but systematic reviews show that both the elderly and women benefit from exercise-based CR (SIGN, 2002; Jolliffe, *et al.*, 2004).

The importance of considering the elderly is even more relevant now, as almost a half of all MIs occur in those over 70 years of age, and this is projected to rise further as the number of older patients in the total population increases (Rask-Madsen, *et al.*, 1997). CR may provide a chance to improve the quality of life in appropriately referred elderly patients. Thow, *et al.* (2000) found that women are poorly represented in CR and suggest that in order to improve uptake and adherence in CR, different strategies, including changes to CR programme structure, gender-specific information, environment and implementing behavioural change, are required to address the specific needs of this group.

In trials of CR the ethnic background of patients is seldom reported, but it is likely that trial participants are mainly white Caucasian, though there is no evidence to suggest that outcomes are less favourable for other ethnic groups (Beswick, *et al.*, 2004). Beswick, *et al.* (2004) further suggest that specific interventions to encourage attendance of these groups could be individualised classes, buddy systems and inclusion in the programme of a significant other. It is generally acknowledged that CR should be all inclusive, with no barriers to inclusion. Strategies should be developed to recruit these previously excluded groups.

CONTENT OF CARDIAC REHABILITATION

Cardiac rehabilitation is a multifaceted intervention offering education, exercise and psychological support for patients with coronary heart disease and their families and involves a variety of specialist health professionals (Bethell, *et al.*, 2001). Cardiac rehabilitation can promote recovery, enable patients to achieve and maintain better health, and reduce the risk of death in people who have heart disease (National Health Service Centre for Reviews and Dissemination, 1998). The challenge of CR, along with all the other aspects of secondary prevention, is the prevention of subsequent cardiovascular events, while maintaining adequate physical functioning and independence and a good quality of life (Giannuzzi, *et al.*, 2003).

Cardiac rehabilitation is a relatively new element in the care of the coronary patient in the UK, first being adopted around the late 1980s (Fearnside, *et al.*, 1999). Cardiac rehabilitation is now embedded as an essential component in the management of heart disease in the UK (Stokes, *et al.*, 1998; Walker, 2003). CR is included in many UK national guidelines and standards. For example,

- British Association for Cardiac Rehabilitation (BACR) Guidelines (BACR, 1995);
- National Service Framework for CHD (Department of Health (DoH), 2000);
- Scottish Intercollegiate Guidelines Network (SIGN, 2002) (endorsed by the BACR, 2003).

All of these have served to add validity to cardiac rehabilitation. These guidelines have been developed over the past ten years, and aim to achieve optimal outcomes for patients with CHD. Cardiac rehabilitation is now 'on the map' and is an established part of cardiac care.

EVIDENCE BASE FOR CARDIAC REHABILITATION

CR has an increasing evidence base as an intervention for secondary prevention (Dalal and Evans, 2003). The focus of research has been primarily in phase III, on post-MI and revascularised patients. The Cochrane review of exercise-based rehabilitation for CHD concluded that exercise-based CR is effective in reducing cardiac deaths, in reducing cardiac risk factors and in enhancing psychosocial factors (Jolliffe, *et al.*, 2004). There is gathering evidence on the impact of CR on many of the newer groups who are being included in CR. A significant feature of CR is that individualised exercise has a positive impact on patients' ability to exercise, on physiological measures of cardiac disease and has not been found to do any harm to patients (Jolliffe, *et al.*, 2004).

There is ample evidence for the later phases of CR. Mayou, *et al.* (2002) comment that there has been surprisingly little clinical and research interest in the earlier stages of the CR programmes, specifically phases I and II. Thus, the evidence base for these phases is less robust.

Benefits of exercise

The benefits of habitual exercise can be viewed as a combination of physiological and psychosocial. In a review of CR post-MI, regular exercise was found to reduce the risk of overall mortality and cardiovascular mortality. In addition, exercise is associated with improved activity tolerance, modification of risk factors and improvement in quality of life (Gassner, *et al.*, 2003).

Physiological Benefits

Physical functioning improves after CR in all age, sex and diagnostic groups, but particularly in patients with low baseline exercise function (McArdle, *et al.*, 2001). For the cardiac patient there are many physiological benefits attributed to exercise training. Many of these changes impart a cardioprotective effect. A study by Leon (2000), reviewing the scientific evidence supporting the potential benefits of exercise post-MI, found the following:

- improvement in functional capacity (strong evidence);
- improved cardiovascular efficiency;
- reduction in atherogenic and thrombotic risk factors;
- improvement in coronary blood flow, reduced myocardial ischaemia and severity of coronary atherosclerosis;
- reduction in risk of cardiovascular disease mortality.

Psychosocial Benefits

Participation in habitual exercise not only has potential impact on physiological function, including reducing cardiac risk factors, but can also aid and enhance psychosocial outcomes. Habitual exercise has potential for the following benefits:

- reduction in depression and anxiety
- enhanced mood status
- enhanced self-efficacy
- restoration of self-confidence
- decreased illness behaviour
- increased social interaction
- resumption of chores/hobbies
- resumption of sexual activities
- return to vocation/work (Ross and Thow, 1997; Goble and Worcester, 1999).

PHASES OF CARDIAC REHABILITATION

Cardiac rehabilitation is divided into four phases, progressing from the acute hospital admission stage to long-term maintenance of lifestyle changes, as follows:

- Phase I – in-patient period or after a 'step change' in cardiac condition;
- Phase II – early post-discharge;
- Phase III – supervised out-patient programme including structured exercise;
- Phase IV – long-term maintenance of exercise and other lifestyle changes.

Phase I cardiac rehabilitation

Phase I, which in most cases is the initial stage of the patient's cardiac rehabilitation pathway, is considered as the in-patient stage, or after a 'step change' in the patient's cardiac condition. These step changes include myocardial infarction, onset of angina, any emergency hospital admission for coronary heart disease, cardiac surgery or angioplasty and/or stent, and first diagnosis of heart failure (SIGN, 2002).

Following an acute coronary event, phase I CR is important in assisting the patient's pathway to recovery. The National Service Framework for CHD (DoH, 2000) states that the aim of this phase is to offer high-quality CR before discharge from hospital, and this should begin as soon as possible after someone is admitted with CHD. Phase I will be the patient's first point of contact with the CR team, and this introduction to CR may favourably or adversely influence their perception of secondary prevention. At this stage, the patient may be anxious and depressed regarding the threat to their health (SIGN, 2002). An important aspect of phase I CR is to allay these fears and promote positive outcomes for both the patient and their significant others (Thompson, 1989).

CONTENT OF PHASE I CARDIAC REHABILITATION

The content of phase I CR has traditionally included assessment, education and exercise/mobilisation. There is an emphasis on reassurance and the positive aspects of recovery post-ACS, revascularisation or other CHD-related admission, specific to each individual. Partners and/or significant others are also involved (SIGN, 2002). Assessment involves identifying risk factors and risk stratification, with the educational aspect providing patients with appropriate individual information regarding CHD, risk factors and lifestyle (BACR, 1995). Mobilisation may include graduated exercise, walking programmes and stair practice.

Assessment and needs

Assessment must be carried out on an individual basis, examining each patient's personal requirements and risk factors and then producing individual tailored plans to meet these needs. The current guidelines (BACR, 1995; DoH, 2000; SIGN, 2002) generally agree that the following are addressed:

- risk stratification and lifestyle modification, as appropriate;
- educational requirements;
- psychological factors, including anxiety and depression;
- needs of significant other(s);
- social, vocational and cultural needs.

Before discharge from hospital patients should be offered, as an integral part of acute care, the following:

- assessment of physical, psychological and social needs for future CR;
- negotiation of a written individual plan for meeting these needs;
- prescription of effective medication, and education about its use, benefits and side effects;
- involvement of relevant informal carer(s);
- provision of information about cardiac support groups;
- provision of locally relevant, written information about CR.

The key elements of phase I include medical evaluation, reassurance, education regarding CHD, correction of cardiac misconceptions, risk factor assessment, mobilisation and discharge planning. In addition, the use of psychological measurement is recommended, using, for example, the hospital anxiety and depression scale (HADS) (Zigmond and Snaith, 1983).

Education

Education is an important element of phase I CR, aiming to decrease the patients' anxiety, and meet the patients' perceived learning needs (Turton, 1998). It should also enable patients to retain the information they are given (Waitkoff and Imburgia, 1990). It is imperative to remember, when working with patients, that each patient is unique, bringing with him or her past experiences, perceptions, coping mechanisms, personalities, support systems, strengths and weaknesses (Robinson, 1999). Thus, appropriate, individualised education is required. The education component should adhere to adult education principles including (SIGN, 2002):

- relevance (tailored to patients' knowledge, beliefs and circumstances);
- feedback (informed regarding progress with learning or change);
- individualisation (tailored to personal needs);
- facilitation (provided with means to take action and/or reduce barriers);
- reinforcement (reward for progress).

In addition, it is recommended that written information is given (SIGN, 2002). This may be, for example, in-house booklets, BHF booklets, or the Heart Manual, which is a comprehensive home-based programme (Lewin, *et al.*, 1992). A patient-held record card or treatment plan is also recommended (BACR, 1995; DoH, 2000).

The content of this part of phase I CR should include educational advice regarding:

- risk factors (modifiable and non-modifiable);
- living with CHD;
- anatomy and physiology of the heart;
- clinical management of CHD;
- cardio-protective diet;
- sensible alcohol use;
- the benefits of exercise;
- cardiac misconceptions;
- return to driving, employment and hobbies;
- holiday advice;
- medications;
- psychological aspects of CHD and stress management;
- sexual activity;
- sleep.

Giannuzzi, *et al.* (2003) examined secondary prevention through CR and suggest much less time is now available to teach the skills required to monitor exercise activity and to cover the other phase I components. With the decreasing length of hospital stay, there is a challenge for health professionals to deliver phase I in shorter periods of time. With short phase I, physiological deconditioning is minimal (Giannuzzi, *et al.*, 2003).

Exercise/mobilisation

The BACR guidelines (BACR, 1995) recommend that patients receive a programme of graduated mobilisation and exercises, so that by discharge time the patient is ambulant, able to climb stairs and attend to his or her own activities of daily living. Individualised home-walking programmes should be prescribed for phase II. Thompson, *et al.* (1996) suggest that prior to discharge, patients are taught simple ways of self-assessing the level of physical activity, using pulse rate measurement and the Borg rating of perceived (RPE) exertion scale (Borg, 1998). Early introduction to the concept and skills of self-monitoring of exercise is important (see Chapter 3). Phase I CR represents for the majority of cardiac patients their first exposure to risk factor modification and education and acts as a gateway to the next phases of CR (Spencer, *et al.*, 2001).

Transition to phase II

It is imperative to optimise the network of care for patients (Robinson, 1999) and to ensure appropriate input from the CR team for each individual prior to discharge and transition to phase II. In addition, prior to discharge it is advantageous to induct and refer patients to phase III CR, for those patients who choose and would benefit from this phase. Exercise consultation and behaviour change strategies are advantageous at this stage to enhance adherence to both lifestyle change and maintenance of exercise in phase II and uptake of phase III in the future (see Chapter 8).

Phase II cardiac rehabilitation

This is the initial post-discharge stage, and can tend to be rather low key, although it is a time when patients may feel isolated and somewhat insecure, and when high levels of anxiety may be present. Thus, it is important that patients and their families/significant others have access to appropriate health care professionals. Depending on the service available, contact with the cardiac rehabilitation team may be by phone or home visit, with primary care also involved. This is the stage where modification of risk factors will start and goals set in phase I CR should start to be realised. For patients issued with the heart manual post-MI, this can be used immediately (Lewin, *et al.*, 1992), and for other patients an individualised walking programme may be started at this stage. The use of pedometers can help patients and CR staff monitor home walking programmes.

Progression to phase III is important, yet despite evidence of the benefits of CR, studies have shown that uptake of the outpatient CR programmes remains low. In a study by Beswick, *et al.* (2004) between 45% and 67% of patients who were referred attended phase III.

For patients who do not proceed to phase III it is important that phase I or II is relevant to and specific for their needs. These patients and families should have information on other sources of support and information on CHD. Health professionals involved in phases I and II need to be aware of the importance of relevant, robust follow-up and of a referral system that enables progress to appropriate, accessible phase III. Utilisation of motivational interviewing and exercise consultation is one method that can be used to influence behaviour change. (See Chapter 8.)

Phase III cardiac rehabilitation

This is traditionally the outpatient education and structured exercise programme component of CR. Phase III continues risk factor changes and education established in previous phases. An individual, menu-based approach continues, with monitoring and feedback regarding risk factors and lifestyle.

There is an emphasis on addressing multi-factorial risk factor modification, appropriate to each patient. Baseline patient assessment can be carried out and outcomes reviewed and audited. Traditionally this phase is hospital-based, though it is increasingly recognised that it can be undertaken safely and successfully in the community (SIGN, 2002). Phase III can also be structured to be sited in the hospital for the first half and in the community for the second half of phase III CR (Armstrong, *et al.*, 2004). This novel design assists patients to enter a community setting where phase IV will be based, thus exposing them to a more social and less medical environment.

The structure of phase III is usually at least two supervised exercise sessions per week, lasting over a period of between 6 and 12 weeks. One session of education per week may be offered. Physical training is often the key component of phase III CR, but psycho-social counselling and education regarding risk factors and lifestyle are important. Strategies to enable a reduction in depression, anxiety and uncertainty, accepting the heart disease and learning to cope with it are discussed as appropriate. As with earlier phases of CR, the involvement of family and significant others continues to be important. Risk stratification prior to patients commencing phase III exercise classes is essential and will be examined in Chapter 2.

In the UK, aerobic circuit interval training for group exercise training is commonly used and is an effective method for delivering aerobic exercise (SIGN, 2002). In addition to the aerobic conditioning phase, resistance training is part of CR exercise. Home-based exercise is also prescribed with self-monitoring skills being used by the patients. Typically an exercise class consists of a warm-up, an aerobic conditioning phase, a cool-down period and a conditioning phase. The exercise programme should be tailored to the needs of the patient. The latter is important to encourage adherence to exercise. Details regarding the exercise component of CR are provided in Chapters 3–5.

Phase IV cardiac rehabilitation

Phase IV CR is the long-term maintenance of risk factor modification, with long-term follow-up in primary care. For the benefits of physical activity and lifestyle change to be sustained, the available evidence suggests that both need to be maintained (SIGN, 2002). As clinically indicated, referral to specialist clinicians, such as smoking cessation or psychological support, may still be required (DoH, 2000). This stage is likely to be the most informal stage of cardiac rehabilitation, where there is long-term maintenance of individual goals and monitoring of clinical issues and risk factor modification, mainly by the primary healthcare team (BACR, 1995). It is important that the patient is aware of the exact nature of the follow-up system available.

Continuation and progression of appropriate physical activities are encouraged outside the hospital setting, on either a formal or informal basis. By this time it is hoped that individuals will be aware of their exercise capabilities and be able to monitor themselves appropriately. The BACR offers a comprehensive training course in phase IV exercise for exercise professionals, such as health and fitness officers who may be involved in community-based programmes.

Phase III discharge information, including goals set, should be sent to the relevant healthcare professional in the community, and formal referral to phase IV exercise classes made. As for earlier phases of CR motivational interviewing and exercise consultation are methods that can be used to maintain behaviour change (see Chapter 8).

SUMMARY

The number and variety of subjects with CHD who are involved in exercise-based CR is increasing. Cardiac rehabilitation is now well established and is part of care of different cardiac groups. There is a growing evidence base for exercise-based CR. There are many benefits for the patient, family and community from regular, long-term participation in CR. The following chapters will address the assessment of the CR participant, design and delivery of the exercise programmes.

REFERENCES

American College of Sports Medicine (2000) *Guidelines for Exercise Testing and Prescription*, 6th edn. Lippincott, Williams and Wilkins, Baltimore, MD.

Armstrong, G., Dunn, M., Bredin, Y., McCuskey, F., Brown, C. (2004) *Patients' Views on Community Cardiac Rehabilitation.* Proceedings of the British Association for Cardiac Rehabilitation Conference.

Beswick, A.D., Rees, K., Griebsch, I., Taylor, F.C., Burke, M., West, R.R., *et al.* (2004) Provision, uptake and cost of cardiac rehabilitation programmes: Improving services to under-represented groups [online] available from http://www.ncchta.org [accessed 19 Nov 2004].

Bethell, H.J.N., Turner, S.C., Evans, J.A., Rose, L. (2001) Cardiac Rehabilitation in the United Kingdom: How complete is the provision? *Journal of Cardiopulmonary Rehabilitation*, **21**, 111–15.

Borg, G.A.V. (1998) *Borg's Perceived Exertion and Pain Scales.* Human Kinetics, London.

British Association for Cardiac Rehabilitation (BACR) (1995) *BACR Guidelines for Cardiac Rehabilitation*, Blackwell Science, Oxford.

British Heart Foundation (BHF) (2003) Coronary heart disease statistics (2003 edn) [online] available from http://www.heartstats.org [accessed 5 Mar 2004].

British Heart Foundation (BHF) (2004) Coronary heart disease statistics (2004 edn) [online] available from http://www.heartstats.org [accessed 18 Sept 2004].

Brugemann, J., Postema, K., van Gelder, I.C., Oosterwijk, M.H., van Veldhuisen, D.J. (2004) Cardiac rehabilitation in patients with a congenital heart disease, an implantable defibrillator or chronic heart failure. *Nederlands Tijdschrift voor Geneeskunde*, **148**(37), 1809–15.

Dalal, H.M., Evans, H. (2003) Achieving national service framework standards for cardiac rehabilitation and secondary prevention. *British Medical Journal*, **326**, 481–4.

Dalal, H., Evans, P.H., Campbell, J.L. (2004) Recent developments in secondary prevention and cardiac rehabilitation after acute myocardial infarction. *British Medical Journal*, **328**, 693–7.

Department of Health (DoH) (2000) National service framework for coronary heart disease modern standards and service models [online] available from http://www.doh.gov.uk/nsf/coronary [accessed 11 Nov 2002].

Durstine, J.L., Moore, G.E. (2003) *ACSM's Exercise Management for Persons with Chronic Diseases and Disabilities*, 2nd edn, Human Kinetics, Leeds.

European Heart Failure Training Group (1998) Experience from controlled trials of physical training in chronic heart failure. *European Heart Journal*, **19**, 466–75.

ExTraMATCH Collaborative (2004) Exercise training meta-analysis of trials in patients with chronic heart failure. *British Medical Journal*, **328**, 189.

Fearnside, E., Hall, S., Lillie, S., Sutcliffe, J., Barrett, J. (1999) Current provision of cardiac rehabilitation in England and Wales. *Coronary Health Care*, **3**, 121–7.

Fitchet, A., Docherty, P.J., Bundy, C., Bell, W., Fitzpatrick, A.P., Garratt, C.J. (2003) Comprehensive cardiac rehabilitation programme for implantable cardioverter defibrillator patients – a randomised controlled trial. *Heart*, **89**(2), 155–60.

Gassner, L-A, Dunn, S., Piller, N. (2003) Aerobic exercise and the post myocardial infarction patient: A review of the literature. *Heart and Lung*, **32**, 258–65.

Giannuzzi, P., Saner, H., Bjornstad, H., Fioretti, P., Mendes, M., Cohen-Solal, A., *et al.* (2003) Secondary prevention through cardiac rehabilitation: Position paper of the working group on cardiac rehabilitation and exercise physiology of the European Society of Cardiology. *European Heart Journal*, **24**, 1273–8.

Goble, A.J., Worcester, M.U.C. (1999) *Best Practice Guidelines for Cardiac Rehabilitation and Secondary Prevention*, The Heart Research Centre, Melbourne.

Imms, C. (2004) Occupational performance challenges for children with congenital heart disease: A literature review. *Canadian Journal of Occupational Therapy*, **71**(3), 161–71.

Jolliffe, J.A., Rees, K., Taylor, R.S., Thompson, D., Oldridge, N., Ebrahim, S. (2004) Exercise-based rehabilitation for coronary heart disease. Cochrane Database for Systematic Reviews.1. [online] available from http://www.cochrane.org [accessed 14 Feb 2004].

Kligfield, P., McCormack, A., Chai, B.S., Jacobson, A., Feuerstadt, B.A., Hao, C. (2003) Effect of age and gender on heart rate recovery after submaximal cardiac rehabilitation in patients with angina pectoris, recent acute myocardial infarction, or coronary bypass surgery. *American Journal of Cardiology*, **5**(1), 600–3.

Kobashigawa, J.A., Leaf, D.A., Lee, N., Gleeson, M.P., Liu, H., Hamilton, M.A., *et al.* (1999) A controlled trial of exercise rehabilitation after heart transplantation. *New England Journal of Medicine*, **340**(4), 272–7.

Leon, A.S. (2000) Exercise following myocardial infarction: Current recommendations. *Sports Medicine*, **29**(5), 301–11.

Leon, A.S., Franklin, B.A., Costa, F., Balady, G.J., Berra, K.A., Stewart, K.J., *et al.* (2005) Cardiac rehabilitation and secondary prevention of coronary heart disease. *Circulation*, **111**, 369–76.

Lewin, B., Robertson, I.H., Cay, E.L., Irving, J.B., Campbell, M. (1992) Effects of self-help post myocardial infarction rehabilitation on psychological adjustment and use of health services. *Lancet*, **339**(1), 1036–40.

Lloyd-Williams, S., Mair, F.S., Lietner, M. (2002) Exercise training and heart failure: A systematic review of current evidence. *British Journal of General Practice*, **January**, 47–55.

Lockhart, L., McMeeken, K., Mark, J., Cross, S., Isles, C. (2000) Secondary prevention after myocardial infarction: Reducing the risk of further cardiovascular events. *Coronary Health Care*, **4**, 82–91.

Mayou, R.A., Thompson, D.R., Clements, A., Davies, C.H., Goowin, S.J., Normington, K., *et al.* (2002) Guideline-based early rehabilitation after myocardial infarction: A pragmatic randomised controlled trial. *Journal of Psychosomatic Research*, **52**, 89–95.

McArdle, W.D., Katch, F.I., Katch, V.L. (2001) *Exercise Physiology: Energy, Nutrition and Human Performance*, 5th edn, Williams and Wilkins, Baltimore, MD.

McKenna, C.J., Forfar, J.C. (2002) Was it a heart attack? *British Medical Journal*, **324**(1), 377–8.

National Centre for Reviews and Dissemination (1998) Cardiac rehabilitation. *Effective Health Care* **4**(4), 1–12.

National Institute for Clinical Excellence (NICE) (2000) Guidance on the use of implantable cardioverter defibrillators for arrhythmias. *NICE Technology Appraisal Guidance*, no. 11, NICE, London.

Rask-Madsen, C., Jensen, G., Kober, L., Melchior, T., Torp-Pedersen, C., Hildebrand, P. (1997) Age-related mortality, clinical heart failure, and ventricular fibrillation in 4259 Danish patients after acute myocardial infarction. *European Heart Journal*, **18**, 1426–31.

Rees, K., Taylor, R.S., Singh, S., Coates, A.J.S., Ebrahim, S. (2004) Exercise based rehabilitation for heart failure. Cochrane Database of Systematic Reviews [online] available from http://www.cochrane.org [accessed 3 February 2005].

Robinson, K.R. (1999) Envisioning a network of care for at-risk patients after myocardial infarction. *Journal of Cardiovascular Nursing*, **14**(1), 75–88.

Ross, A., Thow, M.K. (1997) Exercise as a catalyst. *Coronary Health Care*, **1**(3), 124–9.

Ross, A.B., Brodie, E.E., Carroll, D., Niven, C.A., Hotchkiss, R. (2000) The psychological and physical impact of exercise rehabilitation following coronary artery bypass surgery. *Coronary Health Care*, **4**(2), 63–70.

Santiago, P., Tadros, P. (2002) Non-ST-segment elevation syndromes: pharmacologic management, conservative versus early invasive approach. *Postgraduate Medicine*, **112**(1), 47–68.

Scottish Intercollegiate Guidelines Network (SIGN) (2002) *Cardiac Rehabilitation*, no. 57, Edinburgh.

Shephard, R.J. (1998) How important is exercise-centred rehabilitation following cardiac transplantation? *Critical Reviews in Physical and Rehabilitation Medicine*, **10**(2), 101–21.

Spencer, F.A., Salami, B., Yarzebski, J., Lessard, D., Gore, J.M., Goldberg, R.J. (2001) Temporal trends and associated factors of inpatient cardiac rehabilitation in patients with acute myocardial infarction: A community-wide perspective. *Journal of Cardiopulmonary Rehabilitation*, **21**(6), 377–84.

Stewart, K.J., Badenhop, D., Brubaker, P.H., Keteyian, S.J., King, M. (2003) Cardiac rehabilitation following percutaneous revascularization, heart transplant, heart valve surgery, and for chronic heart failure. *Chest*, **123**, 2104–11.

Stokes, H.C., Thompson, D.R., Seers, K. (1998) The implementation of multiprofessional guidelines for cardiac rehabilitation: A pilot study. *Coronary Health Care*, **2**, 60–71.

Swan, L., Hillis, W.S. (2000) Exercise prescription in adults with congenital heart disease: A long way to go. *Heart*, **83**(6), 685–7.

Taylor, R.S., Brown, A., Ebrahim, S., Jollliffe, J., Noorani, H., Rees, K., *et al.* (2004) Exercise-based rehabilitation for patients with coronary heart disease: systematic review and meta-analysis of randomized trials. *American Medical Journal*, **116**, 682–97.

Thompson, D.R. (1989) A randomized controlled trial of in-hospital nursing support for first time myocardial infarct patients and their partners: Effects on anxiety and depression. *Journal of Advanced Nursing*, **14**, 291–7.

Thompson, D.R., Bowman, G.S., Kitson, A.L., de Bono, D.P., Hopkins, A. (1996) Cardiac rehabilitation in the United Kingdom: Guidelines and audit standards. *Heart*, **75**, 89–93.

Thow, M., Isoud, P., White, M., Robertson, I., Keith, E., Armstrong, G. (2000) Uptake and adherence of women post myocardial infarction to phase III cardiac rehabilitation: Are things changing? *Coronary Health Care*, **4**(4), 174–8.

Todd, I.C., Bradman, M.S., Cooke, M.B., Ballantyne, D. (1991) Effects of daily high-intensity exercise on myocardial perfusion in angina pectoris. *American Journal of Cardiology*, **68**(17), 1593–9.

Turton, J. (1998) Importance of information following myocardial infarction: A study of the self-perceived information needs of patients and their spouse/partner compared with the perceptions of nursing staff. *Journal of Advanced Nursing*, **27**, 770–8.

Vanhees, L., Kornaat, M., Defoor, J., Aufdemkampe, G., Schepers, D., Stevens, A., *et al.* (2004) Effect of exercise training in patients with an implantable cardioverter defibrillator. *European Heart Journal*, **25**(13), 1120–6.

Waitkoff, B., Imburgia, D. (1990) Patient education and continuous improvement in a phase I cardiac rehabilitation program. *Journal of Nursing Quality Assurance*, **5**(1), 38–48.

Walker, J.M. (2003) Rehabilitation: Quantity and quality will count. *British Journal of Cardiology*, **10**, 424–5.

Wanless, D. (2001) Securing our future health: Taking a long-term view, an interim report. [online] available from http://.www.hmtreasury.gov.uk/consultations_and_legislation/wanless/consult_wanles_interimrep.cfm [accessed 20 Feb 2004].

World Health Organisation (1993) *Needs and Action Priorities in Cardiac Rehabilitation and Secondary Prevention in Patients with Coronary Heart Disease*, WHO Regional Office for Europe, Geneva.

Zigmond, A.S., Snaith, R.P. (1983) The hospital anxiety and depression scale. *Acta Psychiatrica Scandinavica*, **67**, 361–7.

Chapter 2

Risk Stratification and Health Screening for Exercise in Cardiac Rehabilitation

Ann Ross and Mhairi Campbell

Chapter outline

The previous chapter has provided an overview of the content and background to Cardiac Rehabilitation CR within the UK context. The aim of this chapter is to highlight available evidence and/or the rationale for the risk stratification and health screening process, as currently applied. In addition, it directs the CR practitioner to reflect on current practice in risk stratification for CR exercise.

APPROACH TO RISK STRATIFICATION

In this chapter we deliberate over current patient assessment procedures for entry into CR programmes. We do not attempt to describe the ultimate blueprint for the risk stratification and assessment of patients for the exercise component. Nonetheless, we discuss current accepted practice and explore the evidence to support it. In addition, we will describe a fresh approach proposed by the Canadian Association of Cardiac Rehabilitation (Stone, *et al.*, 2001) for effectively determining a patient's risk of exercise-related cardiac events. The chapter will explore the variety of different processes and approaches used to understand assessment and risk stratification and the characteristics of each including pros and cons.

Exercise Leadership in Cardiac Rehabilitation. An Evidence-Based Approach. Edited by Morag Thow.
Copyright 2006 by John Wiley & Sons Ltd. ISBN 0-470-01971-9

Risk stratification can be considered as the crux of assessment prior to entry into CR, but this approach should form part of a process of sound clinical reasoning. The reader will find reference to commonly used coronary heart disease (CHD) risk-stratification guidelines for supervised exercise. These guidelines are produced by authoritative organisations well respected in this field – American Heart Association (AHA, 2001), SIGN (2002) and the American Association of Cardiovascular and Pulmonary Rehabilitation (AACVPR, 2004).

DEFINITION OF RISK STRATIFICATION

When using the term 'risk stratification', it becomes apparent that for CR professionals the concept is very different from that used by those concerned with the medical management of CHD patients. In medical practice the physician or health practitioner considers quantifying the risk of CHD for an individual either in terms of absolute or relative risk. Absolute risk relates to a specific 'risky behaviour' where statistics define the risk within a population. Relative risk relates risk to an individual and compares that person's risk within a specific group, i.e. same age/gender and expresses this as a ratio (Lindsay, 2004).

Both approaches are useful predictors in the primary care (PC) setting for CHD prevention and effective medical management. In secondary prevention (SP), the physician or health practitioner deliberates the likelihood of recurrent cardiac events in relation to disease prognosis and progression. Ultimately this determines ongoing medical intervention.

The purpose of risk stratification in CHD medical management, therefore, is to identify those most at risk of developing CHD and/or from subsequent cardiac events in order to instigate optimum medical management. In the CR setting, however, the aim is to attempt to predict those at risk of exercise-related cardiac incidents and to tailor exercise prescription, supervision and monitoring appropriately to the individual.

EXERCISE IN CORONARY HEART DISEASE PREVENTION

Strong evidence exists to support the view that the health and fitness benefits of physical activity have a direct dose–response relationship. Public health messages worldwide advocate the need for the general public to take up at least moderate amounts of physical activity. Extensive research has demonstrated that the benefits related to exercise training are also afforded to patients with demonstrable cardiovascular disease (see Chapter 1).

CHD continues to be the foremost cause of death in both men and women in the UK, European Union and USA and, in addition, the numbers of patients surviving coronary events are escalating year on year. Although we all recognise the importance of primary prevention of CHD, there is no question that the role of CR is pivotal as a secondary prevention intervention, a concept recognised by numerous countries throughout the world as extremely important. Policy statements and practice guidelines across the UK, USA, Europe and Australia all advocate that comprehensive CR should be available to all patients with cardiac and vascular disease.

As treatment options for the post-myocardial infarction (MI) patient have developed, there has been a resulting improvement in survival rates. As a result there have been both changes in the demographics, i.e. diagnosis of patients eligible, and an increase in the number of patients referred to CR.

It is imperative, therefore, that the exercise professional recognises the likelihood of exercise-related incidents and takes all reasonable steps to ensure safe and effective exercise prescription for those individuals with diagnosed CHD.

EXERCISING THE CHD PATIENT: THE NEED FOR ASSESSMENT AND RISK STRATIFICATION

Exercise training in individuals with CHD has been the subject of numerous clinical trials, with the evidence strongly demonstrating that exercise-based cardiac rehabilitation is associated with a reduction in coronary mortality and morbidity. Early trials supporting this evidence by Oldridge, *et al.* (1988) and O'Connor, *et al.* (1989) have more recently been confirmed by SIGN (2002) and Jolliffe, *et al.* (2004). This supports the premise that the benefits outweigh the risks. Despite the low incidence of adverse events, most international CR guidelines, nevertheless, recommend that, prior to recruitment to the exercise programme, patients should undergo a comprehensive assessment, including risk stratification.

Although the data would suggest that the increased myocardial demands of vigorous exercise may precipitate cardiovascular events, i.e. ventricular fibrillation, the evidence indicates that mortality is lowest in those who are physically active. The risk of cardiac events during exercise is small, particularly where evidence of substantial cardiac disease is absent. Within supervised CR programmes the risk of serious exercise-related cardiac events is also small, with evidence from Paul-Labrador, *et al.* (1999) suggesting that it is approximately 50% of the incidence observed in joggers than in the general public (1 in 784 000 versus 1 in 396 000 respectively).

Verrill, *et al.* (1996) reviewed the literature to ascertain the occurrence of cardiac arrest during CR exercise programmes. At their cardiopulmonary research institute there were 25 cardiac arrests between 1968 and 1981 (374, 616 hrs), nine of which occurred during the 'cool-down' period. The significance of this finding will be discussed further in Chapter 6.

Additionally, Vongvanich, *et al.* (1996) carried out a survey to determine the safety of medically supervised rehabilitation and confirmed that event rates are indeed low.

Incidents are most likely in the following categories:

- patients with marked ST-segment depression on ECG;
- patients with an above average exercise capacity;
- patients who have shown poor compliance to exercise intensity guidelines.

There is, however, little recent data that reflect the complexity and varied risk of exercise-related events for the patient group now eligible for CR. In addition, most of the available data are from the United States, where electrocardiogram (ECG) monitoring and trans-telephonic monitoring are standard, making it difficult to generalise this to other healthcare systems, where appropriate professional supervision is the predominant monitoring tool. In addition, Paul-Labrador, *et al.* (1999) concluded that contemporary American CR guidelines did not accurately predict complications during exercise. However, adverse events remained consistent with the 1970s data, suggesting that there was a trade-off between the general lowering of risk achieved by developments in treatment and medications and an increase in risk with the inclusion of more complex and older patients in CR exercise.

THE PROCESS OF RISK STRATIFICATION

The purpose of the risk-stratification process is to identify all the factors related to an individual and place them in a risk category based on an increased likelihood of adverse effects. This provides the exercise leader with guidance in respect to exercise prescription, monitoring and supervision. Most risk-stratification tools classify individuals into low, medium/moderate and high risk categories. However, at this time, there would appear to be no clearly validated comprehensive risk-assessment tool for entry to the exercise component of CR. All international guidelines for CR nevertheless advocate a similar approach. Table 2.1 shows the AACVPR (2004) guidelines. Individuals who do not meet the classification for either low or high are defined as moderate or medium risk.

The summary of the 1999 Canadian Guidelines (Stone, *et al.*, 2001) has, however, proposed three possible strategies for the risk stratification of patients entering CR programmes. One approach is based on the long-standing, traditional format, established by the AHA (2001) and the AACVPR (2004) and which classifies risk stratification into low (class A), intermediate (class B) and high risk (class C) categories. This system has been adopted by most CR professionals to date. However, it is an approach which seems to reflect sound medical judgement and evidence-based practice, but fails to take

Table 2.1. Characteristics of low and high risk CR
(Adapted from the AACPR, 2004)

A low-risk individual would have *all* of the following:	A high-risk individual would have only *one* of the following:
Normal haemodynamic response to exercise and recovery	Decreased left ventricular function – ejection fraction <40%
No evidence of myocardial ischaemia	Abnormal haemodynamic response with exercise and recovery
Normal left ventricular function	Persistent or recurrent ischaemia at low levels of exercise
Functional capacity of 7 METs (metabolic equivalents) or more	Functional capacity of <5 METs
Absence of clinical depression	Survivor of cardiac arrest or sudden death
	Complicated recovery post-event, i.e. cardiogenic shock, CHF
	Clinically significant depression

Box 2.1 Discussion point on risk stratification

Discussion point:

Is it perhaps time for CR professionals to look at current practice of risk stratification and to consider how risky behaviours, e.g. smoking, have an indirect effect on risk during exercise corresponding to plaque stability?

Paul-Labrador, *et al.* (1999) proposed that the risk shifts over time, the risk being related to the atherosclerotic plaque stability, and suggests that perhaps our initial risk assessment should be revisited regularly and risk stratification performed at regular intervals in relation to disease stability. Angioplasty patients, for example, are currently considered by many to be low risk, but Paul-Labrador, *et al.* (1999) found in their survey that this patient group had more complications than the post-MI or bypass patients.

account of the individuals' other health behaviour and motivational risk factors. This is an issue which often leads to confusion, particularly where in primary prevention the focus is on lifestyle issues like smoking and the recognised risk markers for CHD, e.g. hypertension. Box 2.1 poses this question.

The second Canadian Guideline (Stone, *et al.*, 2001) proposal is to use a risk-stratification tool which analyses the risk of subsequent cardiac events (exercise-related) and the risk of disease progression, as directed by the presence and severity of the individual's risk markers. The third Canadian Guideline (Stone, *et al.*, 2001) proposal is to merge the Duke Treadmill score, CCS (Canadian Cardiovascular Society) class score (Campeau, 1976) and the

NYHA (New York Heart Association, 1994) scores. However, although these are three validated tools they have not been validated for use together.

The second Canadian Guideline proposal is worth exploring, as it may give the clinician a more standardised method of risk stratification. It takes the process of risk stratification a stage further, using a scale that generates a score. Additionally, long-term progression risk is taken into account, where the presence and severity of modifiable risk markers are considered. This risk marker score is used in conjunction with the acute risk score giving a quantifiable indication of overall risk.

This would appear to be the first novel approach which attempts to develop a measurable risk-stratification process. In practice, this method would support the approach taken by most CR exercise leaders, where experienced professionals utilise their knowledge, experience and expert judgement to determine both the exercise prescription and appropriate monitoring of individuals within the CR programme. In addition, the approach where other health behaviours are integrated into risk stratification is worth considering. However, the Canadian Association of Cardiac Rehabilitation recently published a second edition of their Guidelines (Stone, *et al.*, 2005). They continue to advocate the use of key principles:

- matching the degree of intervention to the degree of risk;
- recognising that the risk factor burden increases the likelihood of atherosclerotic progression;
- recognising that the likelihood of exercise-related adverse events relates to functional capacity, left ventricular function, ischaemic burden and dysrhythmic monitoring.

However, they have revised their 1999 proposed system for predicting exercise-related adverse events and acknowledge that programmes encounter logistical problems gaining the required objective information. They have concentrated on determination of functional capacity by use of stress testing as the most practical marker for event prediction.

This serves to highlight the difficulty in establishing a comprehensive, user-friendly model of risk stratification which can be applied by the majority of programmes.

The scenario in Table 2.2 highlights the complexity of implementing risk stratification within the cardiac rehabilitation setting as highlighted by the evidence within this chapter. This individual shows the difficulty of 'ticking a box' in relation to risk stratification and how there is an ever-changing picture that takes into consideration all the factors discussed in the chapter and the use of skilled clinical judgement that informs individualised care packages that offer a menu of services and advice.

Table 2.2. A scenario of a young cardiac rehabilitation patient showing the complexity and changing picture of medical markers, health behaviour and motivational risk factors

	Key Characteristics
Time-point 1 (initial event)	• 47-year-old man • Non-ST elevation MI • First cardiac event • Good LV function on echocardiography • Modified Bruce pre-discharge ETT: 4.6 ml.kg^{-1}.min^{-1} METs limited by chest pain and max ST depression of –1.75 mm in anterior leads. • Pain ongoing after ETT – sent for angiography
Time-point 2 (pre-phase III)	• Returns post-PTCA to single lesion in mid-LAD • Asymptomatic • Stopped smoking • Completes SWT with estimated MET value of 9.1 ml.kg^{-1}.min^{-1}
Time-point 3 (during course of phase III)	• Non-compliance with given exercise prescription • Exceeds target heart rate • Increases exercise intensity independently • Unable to use perceived exertion scale as underestimates own exertion levels • Demonstrates hostility towards staff who try to advise re-modification of exercise behaviour • Competitive with other patients
Time-point 4 (phase III completion)	• Still lacks self-monitoring skills • Anxiety and depression scale now indicates borderline depression • Altered sleep pattern • Atypical chest pain • Recommenced smoking

COMPONENTS OF RISK STRATIFICATION

Irrespective of which tool is adopted, consensus would advocate that the key aspects that should be considered in the risk stratification process are:

- Functional capacity.
- Ischaemic burden (myocardial ischaemia).
- Arrhythmic potential.
- Left ventricular function.

Although these aspects can be considered individually, they are very much interrelated. The following section reviews each.

Functional capacity

Functional capacity has been reported to be a powerful prognostic indicator (Chang and Froelicher, 1994; Myers, *et al.*, 2000; Kavanagh, *et al.*, 2002). Kavanagh, *et al.* (2002) analysed data in an extensive cohort of 12 169 male coronary patients, and Myers, *et al.* (2002) studied 6213 men.

In both studies, in individuals both with and without CHD, peak exercise capacity was shown to be the most important predictor of prognosis and risk of subsequent death, having greater significance than other risk factors, such as smoking, diabetes and hypertension. Myers, *et al.* (2002) also found it to be a stronger predictor than other measures recorded during an exercise test, e.g. arrhythmia, ST-segment depression or peak heart rate.

A one MET (metabolic equivalents $3.5 \, \text{ml.kg}^{-1}.\text{min}^{-1}$) increase in exercise capacity (peak VO_2) can improve survival by 12% (Myers, *et al.*, 2002), and an even more modest $1 \, \text{ml.kg}^{-1}.\text{min}^{-1}$ (0.28 of a MET) can improve survival by 9% (Kavanagh, *et al.*, 2002).

In a 1991 review of the literature, Morris, *et al.* (1991) concluded that an exercise capacity of <6 METs indicates higher mortality, a theory also advocated by the 'big four' American Associations in their risk tables. Myers, *et al.* (2002) found that 5 METs distinguished between better and poorer survival rates, with those at <5 METs being at double the risk of all-cause mortality than those with >8 METs.

The majority of the studies reviewed by Morris, *et al.* (1991) made no adjustment for other factors which may have a direct bearing on exercise capacity, including the influence of non-cardiac co-morbidity on mortality.

Nonetheless, exercise capacity has shown itself to be clinically significant, and should be a core component of both the pre- and post-rehabilitation assessment (ACPICR, 1999; SIGN, 2002).

Measurement of functional capacity

Exercise tolerance testing (ETT), or field tests of functional capacity, can produce an estimated METs value to guide risk stratification and exercise prescription. True values can only be obtained through cardio-pulmonary exercise testing using gas analysis. Predicted VO_2max or extrapolated MET values have a degree of error, as compared to true VO_2max when measured using gas analysis.

Factors Influencing Accuracy in Clinical Practice (METs or VO_2MAX/PEAK)

- The use of a sub-maximal symptom limited test:
  A sub-maximal test is thought to give a measurement within 10–20% of a normal individual's actual VO_2max. These tests are often used in pre-discharge evaluation of post-MI patients (ACSM, 2001). In relation to a

clinical population, symptom-limited testing is probably the most appropriate, as any exercise prescriptions should be based on what actually limits the patient.

- The most widely used ETT protocol is the Bruce treadmill protocol (ACSM, 2001) with a recent survey showing that 82% of treadmill tests in America used either the Bruce or modified Bruce (Myers, *et al.*, 2000). The METs levels associated with each increment of the test were developed from early research on healthy subjects, of a younger age than the clinical population and on the assumption of reaching steady state exercise within the three-minute, large incremental increases in workload (ACSM, 2001; AHA, 2001).
- The use of age-adjusted predicted maximum heart rates:
  There is a +/− 10 bpm standard deviation in individual maximum heart rate (Balady and Donald, 1991; AHA, 2001; McArdle, *et al.*, 2001).
- An assumed efficiency or economy of task performance:
  This is applicable to the Bruce protocol where METs are estimated from the applied workload or in the shuttle walk test where estimated METs levels are associated with a particular speed of walking. This is also illustrated by evidence that the use of handrails during treadmill testing can reduce the energy cost by 30% and would underestimate an individual's true exercise capacity (McArdle, *et al.*, 2001). Another example is patients with significant co-morbidities, e.g. peripheral vascular disease or osteoarthritis. These patents are potentially working at a higher percentage of their VO_2max at a set pace on incremental treadmill tests to archive the workload. This could lead to over-prescription for their CR exercise intensity.
- Psychological and motivational factors may also contribute to the accuracy of functional capacity measurement. This is an important consideration in the CR population, where levels of anxiety may be high. Individuals are less likely to be familiar with either performing strenuous exercise or with the associated sensations and possible discomfort (McArdle, *et al.*, 2001). This may, therefore, result in an underestimation of true exercise capacity potential (ACSM, 2001). Conversely, trained individuals are more likely to be motivated, confident and able to push themselves into anaerobic exercise and closer to true VO_2max.

There are, therefore, many factors that can affect the accuracy of determining METs, peak or VO_2max; both under-estimation and over-estimation are possible, depending on the patient. We concur with other texts (ACSM, 2001; AHA, 2001; McArdle, *et al.*, 2001) that accept that these errors exist, but for the purposes of risk stratification in a clinical setting such as CR, the most commonly practised methods of estimating METs or VO_2 give a sufficiently accurate indication of exercise capacity.

Most clinical guidelines (ACPICR, 1999; Goble and Worcester, 1999; SIGN, 2002) recommend the inclusion of a measure of exercise tolerance (e.g. treadmill or cycle ergometer testing, shuttle walk test or six-minute walking test) prior to programme commencement in order to allow appropriate stratification and prescription of an individualised exercise programme. Repeated post-rehabilitation testing by the clinical exercise leader allows an increase in exercise capacity to be quantified, supplying an outcome measure for exercise intervention within local programmes.

One of the most commonly used and cardiac population validated tests is the shuttle walking test (SWT) first described by Singh, *et al.* (1992) and used for measurement of functional capacity (Tobin and Thow, 1999). A protocol for implementation of the SWT is included in the SIGN guideline 57 (2002) along with information as to how the test can be purchased (see Chapter 3). It is simple to use, requires little equipment and can be undertaken by the majority of cardiac patients. A study by Fowler, *et al.* (2005) of 39 CABG patients found the SWT was reproducible and sensitive to change. The authors suggest one practice walk for the SWT. None of the 39 subjects in Fowler, *et al.*'s (2005) study completed the entire 12-level protocol. The SWT does, however, have limitations for a small number of patients, who may have a higher baseline fitness level. These patients will 'top out', i.e. they will reach the end of the test protocol before reaching their termination point. The SWT has an estimated top energy expenditure of 9.1 METs, with a maximum walking/running speed of 8.53 km/hour. This leaves the practitioner unable to measure improvement in this small number of patients post-rehabilitation (Armstrong, 2005).

In addition, the ageing population of cardiac rehabilitation patients, with numerous co-morbidities, may find the SWT less sensitive to change when measurement of improved aerobic capacity cannot be demonstrated by incremental walking. A six-minute walking test (Demers, *et al.*, 2001) or other functional outcome measures currently used in elderly rehabilitation may be more sensitive to change, and also more relevant to patient goals in the older population (e.g. functional reach). These examples highlight the importance, when dealing with such a varied group of patients, of having a variety of outcome measures to suit both the patients' abilities and their goals (see Chapter 3 for more on functional capacity).

Ischaemic burden (myocardial ischaemia)

The presence of ischaemia during exercise can be explained in terms of physiological response. As an individual steps up his or her level of activity, myocardial oxygen consumption rises (Rate Pressure Product (RPP) = HR × SBP). Simultaneously, there is a shortening of diastole and subsequently a decrease in coronary perfusion time. Consequently, there is a transient oxygen deficiency to the myocardium. Myocardium deprived of oxygen is unable to meet the demand of the increased activity, and the individual complains of angina, or ST depression is identified on the ECG.

From the clinician's perspective the outcome may be that the patient develops life-threatening electrical disturbances. As the exercise level increases, the resulting increased sympathetic activity leads to an alteration in the depolarization/repolarisation mechanism, with resulting distortion in the conduction velocity. This may give rise to increased ventricular ectopic activity and potentially ventricular tachycardia and/or fibrillation. The degree of ischaemia present and the workload at which this occurs is of enormous importance to the exercise leader. This information will guide the exercise prescription of the individual or ultimately determine entry to the exercise component of CR.

To establish the ischaemic burden or degree of myocardial ischaemia in an individual patient, the CR professional can refer to both technological and clinical examination of the patient. A clinical history of angina, relieved by rest and/or GTN spray, can help the exercise professional classify the individual. A dialogue about the precipitation of chest pain in relation to everyday activities can direct the exercise professional to the level of prescription required to work beneath the ischaemic threshold.

Stress testing can elicit ischaemic changes, revealing ST segment changes and/or myocardial perfusion rates. In general terms, ST displacement of 1–2 mm would be considered as confirmation of moderate myocardial ischaemia, with anything greater that 2 mm regarded as significant. Patients with ischaemia on ECG, or angina at a low workload have a poorer prognosis. This is in line with previous trials (Jesperson, *et al.*, 1993) where a positive test doubles the risk of reinfarction and death in the short to medium term and early ST-segment depression of >2 mm increases the risk of an unfavourable conclusion. They conclude that symptomatic exercise-induced angina at a low workload were independent predictors of mortality with a relative risk of 2.07 and 1.78 respectively. Studies of perfusion abnormalities similarly would consider that the magnitude of the abnormality is the single most effective prognostic indicator of risk, with those patients with mildly abnormal single photon emission computed tomography (SPECT) scan after ETT being in a low-risk category of cardiac death but intermediate risk of non-fatal MI. Conversely, those with extensive scan abnormalities have significant risk of cardiac death (Hachamovitch, *et al.*, 1998).

Occasionally these ischaemic changes may be established from ambulatory, 24 hr Holter monitoring. These data are particularly useful in those individuals with 'silent ischaemia', i.e. absence of pain. Silent ischaemia has been found to occur in 2.5% of the male population (McMurray and Stewart, 2000) and represents impaired myocardial perfusion. A number of patients, diabetics especially, may have silent ischaemia. This can present the exercise professional with an additional challenge when risk stratifying and prescribing exercise, unless information on ischaemic threshold is available. In general, the greater degree of ST depression, the greater the likelihood of the patient experiencing chest pain.

Arrhythmic potential

The increase in myocardial oxygen consumption associated with vigorous activity, and the corresponding decrease in coronary perfusion time, can result in a temporary deficit of oxygen to the myocardium. At the same time the effect of the increased workload results in an increase in circulating catecholamines, with an alteration in the sodium–potassium balance that results in an increased myocardial irritability and produces amplified ventricular activity (ACSM, 2001). It is important to establish the level of arrhythmia production, in particular ventricular tachycardia (subsequently associated with ventricular fibrillation), prior to entry into CR. This can be gained from either an ETT or through 24-hour ambulatory monitoring. However, careful interpretation is required, as a single occurrence of ventricular tachycardia during a stress test is not necessarily an indication of the onset of fatal ventricular fibrillation. Nevertheless, it should be highlighted that an individual who has experienced an episode of ventricular fibrillation (VF) that did not occur in the presence of an acute event or cardiac procedure would be considered moderate to high risk (AHA, 2001). Similarly ventricular arrhythmias (VA) which are uncontrolled at low to moderate workloads with medication would be considered at greater risk for cardiac-related complications during exercise.

Those at greatest risk of exercise-induced ventricular fibrillation are individuals with significantly impaired left ventricular function: namely those who have serious/major myocardial damage, due either to a large infarct, multiple infarctions or other conditions affecting ventricular function, e.g. valve disease, myocarditis, hypertension and cardiomyopathy. There is a lack of recent evidence on the incidence of arrhythmic events during CR. In a study cited by Belardinelli (2003) a programme of exercise training for heart failure patients had only one episode of cardiac arrest in 16 years, i.e. 1 per 130 000 patient hours. However, as Belardinelli (2003) suggests, the low incidence of arrhythmia, as with other complications, during CR is because exercise is safe if the exercise prescription is 'tailored to the patient's clinical picture and needs'.

Left ventricular function

It is generally accepted that impairment of left ventricular (LV) function is a strong predictor of prognosis, with a number of authors rating it as the most powerful predictor (Specchia, *et al.*, 1996). The most widely practised method of assessing LV function is echocardiography. LV function can be expressed as a verbal description, as an ejection fraction (%) or wall motion index. Although less common, LV function can also be assessed during angiography or perfusion scanning. Although ejection fraction as a percentage is less commonly available to exercise practitioners, it is accepted that normal ejection fraction approximates to 60–70%. Variations exist within the literature as to clearly defined links between ejection fraction percentages, verbal descriptors

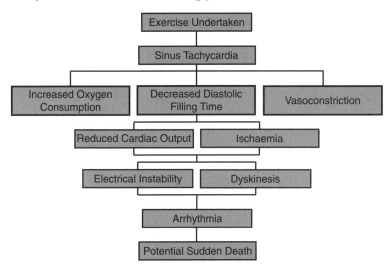

Figure 2.1. Possible adverse physiological consequences of exercise in presence of heart failure (Adapted from Belardinelli, 2003).

and level of risk. Some of the risk table summary data report that only at the level of poor LV function is this considered a high risk variable (Paul-Labrador, *et al.*, 1999). However, the Canadian guidelines (Stone, *et al.*, 2001) classify high risk as <40%, moderate as >40%, and low risk as >50%.

In relation to risk stratification for exercise, LV dysfunction is an indicator of increased risk of complication during exercise. Figure 2.1 illustrates a proposed physiological response to exercise in the presence of heart failure. This explains the link between exercise and adverse event in individuals with impaired LV function.

This figure shows that the sequence of events links LV dysfunction directly to other components of risk stratification already discussed, namely, arrhythmic potential and exercise capacity, due to compromised cardiac output and ischaemic burden.

The information the exercise professional can gather regarding LV function will be relevant for only a specific time. Predicted spontaneous recovery and pharmaceutical interventions (especially ACE inhibition) may have an effect on LV function between time of event and commencement of phase III exercise. Contrary to historical evidence, which suggested LV-impaired patients could not increase cardiac output sufficiently to benefit from rehabilitation, recent research shows that exercise training itself improves survival in the presence of LV dysfunction (Specchia, *et al.*, 1996). Goebbels, *et al.* (1998) conducted a randomised controlled trial that showed a more favourable benefit from exercise rehabilitation for those with reduced ejection fractions (<40%).

EXERCISE PROGRAMME

Numerous patients are enrolled into CR programmes each week, and the vast majority will undertake their exercise prescription without any adverse event. This is mainly due to the effective pre-entry screening, knowledge and skills of the CR professionals in these patient services.

Historically, CR programmes were delivered in the outpatient areas of local hospitals, but now it is common for the exercise component to be delivered in fitness centres, health centres and community halls, thus improving access. The literature indicates that low to moderate intensity exercise for low to moderate risk patients can be delivered safely in the community (Armstrong, *et al.*, 2004). However, patients deemed to be high risk or undertaking high intensity exercise should be limited to hospital-based programmes, supervised by appropriately trained and experienced health professionals (Stone, *et al.*, 2001) and where full resuscitation facilities are available (SIGN, 2002).

CR professionals would concur that, as far as possible, patients should not be excluded from CR and exercise prescription should be a component of that service. Suggested exclusion criteria from Balady and Donald (1991), ACSM (1995), BACR (1995) and Goble and Worcester (1999) are shown below in Table 2.3. Many of these patients can safely enter exercise-based CR when these exclusion criteria are stabilised.

COMPONENTS OF CLINICAL ASSESSMENT

The following section details key components of a pre-exercise assessment, but is by no means exhaustive. It describes the rationale for each component, including supporting evidence, and highlights links to the risk categories previously detailed, i.e. functional capacity, ischaemic burden, arrhythmic potential and LV function.

Assessment of the patient should include not only the risk-stratification process and establishment of functional capacity; there should also be a gathering of further information during a subjective interview.

This assessment process may take place repeatedly over the four phases of rehabilitation, with a number of factors being assessed in phase I and re-assessed over time. This will give a holistic view of the patient, highlighting factors, which may influence progress, adherence or long-term behaviour change, e.g. co-morbidities, stage of change and quality of life (as seen in Table 2.2).

For patients who are unable to undertake exercise testing or for clinicians who do not have access to resources or facilities for functional capacity testing, this assessment becomes the risk-stratification tool itself. This type of holistic assessment has been developed by individual expert practitioners and refined as the specialty of CR has evolved over the last 20 years. It highlights the

Table 2.3. Exclusion criteria for exercise-based CR

Exclusion Criteria	ACSM 2001	Goble and Worcester 1999	BACR 1995	Balady and Donald 1991
Unstable angina	✓	✓	✓	✓
Resting BP >200 systolic or >110/110 diastolic	✓	✓	✓	✓
Significant aortic stenosis	✓	✓	✓	✓
Orthostatic hypotension	✓	✓	✓	
Acute illness or fever/viral infection	✓	✓	✓	
Active peri/myocarditis	✓	✓	✓	✓
New or uncontrolled tachycardia >120	✓	✓	✓ –100 bpm	
Uncompensated HF	✓	✓		✓
New or uncontrolled arrhythmias – a or v or 3rd degree block	✓	✓	✓	✓
Uncontrolled diabetes or metabolic disturbance	✓	✓		
Severe co-morbidity preventing participation – physical or psychological	✓	✓		
Recent pulmonary or other embolism	✓	✓		
Resting ST-segment displacement 2 mm	✓			
Recent stroke, TIA		✓		
Patient or physician refusal		✓		
New or recent breathlessness, palpitations, dizziness or lethargy			✓	
Hypertrophic cardiomyopathy			✓	✓

importance of high-level clinical reasoning skills (Castle, 2003) in the exercise professional and of his or her ability to apply clinical judgement to each patient.

There are numerous patient-related factors that can be included in a comprehensive multidisciplinary assessment (e.g. social support, anxiety and depression, smoking status, age, gender, etc.) of that, although not directly related to risk stratification or assessment for exercise, can have a significant effect on patient adherence or progress within a CR programme.

Prior to meeting the patient the exercise leader must ascertain the current referral for cardiac rehabilitation and exercise assessment. As the eligibility of patients with CHD has widened from post-MI and post-CABG, not all patients will undergo medical investigation prior to CR programme entry. For example, many revascularisation patients no longer have routine ETT, and it is unlikely that angina patients will receive echocardiography. The clinician, therefore, has to look for historical information to create a picture of what the ischaemic burden, arrhythmic potential and LV function may be. Key indicators would be:

- previous MIs
- site and size of infarct
- enzyme results
- thrombolysis with ECG resolution or not
- complication during phase I, i.e. cardiogenic shock, cardiac arrest
- complicated abnormal resting ECG
- site and severity of lesions from angiography
- potential for revascularisation of lesion
- history of AF.

Symptoms

A detailed subjective assessment of symptoms can be an invaluable tool for the CR clinician, even in the absence of more accurate scientific risk stratification data. A patient describing nocturnal or resting symptoms will be a significant characteristic. Establishing a baseline pattern of cardiac-related symptoms could include questions on:

- frequency
- intensity
- duration
- trigger factors, e.g. level of exertion, specific daily activities, stress or emotion
- use of nitrate
- typical versus non-typical patterns of symptoms
- simple description of site and type of pain
- ability to recognise and manage symptoms or absence of symptoms.

Gathering all this information gives the CR exercise leader and CR team an initial indication of physical and psychological functioning, and of whether symptoms are likely to be a limiting factor. It also enables comparison of these factors pre- and post-rehabilitation, by which time the patient may have learnt to manage symptoms more effectively, have gained confidence and improved level of function.

Within the context of risk stratification, assessing cardiac symptoms directly links the ischaemic burden and functional capacity, if the patient can describe a level of exertion required to bring on symptoms. However, it must be remembered that the relationship between symptoms, functional ability and disease severity is complex; patients with the most severe disease do not always demonstrate the most limitation or disability. Lewin (1997) suggests that other factors, such as health beliefs, anxiety and depression, personality, social support, social class and the patient's own attempts to cope will influence the level of disability demonstrated (see more in Chapter 8).

OCCUPATION

Return to work is an important measure of successful CR for some individuals with CHD. Variables which contribute to a successful return to employment or being considered fit to work include shift patterns, self-efficacy, perception of control over work demands and physical job requirements (ACSM, 2001).

The process of assessment for exercise, the consequent advice and guidance, and the exercise prescription itself should contribute to a tailored return to work needs for appropriate patients. These discussions to establish realistic return to work plans should commence as early as possible in the rehabilitation process. The aims of the occupational assessment are:

- discuss job demands (physical and psychological) and concerns;
- provide provisional timelines for return to work based on job analysis;
- provide an individualised exercise prescription based on job analysis;
- consider whether specific occupational carrying or lifting tests should be used for prescription.

(Adapted from ACSM, 2001).

Occupation, work conditions and demands may also impact on patients' ability to commit to attending cardiac rehabilitation programmes. The clinician may need to consider adapting supervised sessions or creating flexibility within programmes to accommodate work commitments, or to involve, where possible, not only the patient but the employer or occupational health representative in planning a rehabilitation programme.

When considering occupation, level of physical effort, including arm versus leg work, carrying and lifting activities, sustained versus bouts of exertion and environmental conditions could influence the type of exercise prescribed for assisting return to work. Driving occupations often require re-licensing using strict criteria on ETT (DVLA, 2004). The CR clinician can use assessment information and rehabilitation to prepare the patient for ETT requirements or to ascertain whether attainment of the level of functional capacity required for re-licensing is realistic for that individual. A detailed discussion around occupation at baseline assessment will reveal whether the patient considers himself or herself ready for return to work. This discussion is important when setting and working towards patient-centred goals. Despite many patients reporting that their jobs are physically active, most occupations require an energy expenditure of less than 5 METs (ACSM, 2001).

PREVIOUS MEDICAL HISTORY AND CO-MORBIDITY

This is possibly the most important non-CHD assessment factor that influences exercise prescription in CR. As the patient population within phase III cardiac rehabilitation expanded and became more inclusive for those with more limited exercise ability, either through age or complex medical history, so our assessment had to expand to consider a diverse and substantial number and combination of orthopaedic, neurological, respiratory, vascular and musculoskeletal conditions. A survey carried out by Thow, *et al.* (2003) looked at non-cardiac patient interventions within eight cardiac rehabilitation programmes in the West of Scotland. Of the 701 interventions carried out over a two-month period, 72% of these were to adapt exercise programmes in light of non-cardiac conditions or to give advice on the same. This highlights the importance both of individualising exercise prescription in the presence of co-morbidity and of having suitably trained exercise professionals to assess, advise patients and deliver phase III cardiac rehabilitation.

The increase in participants with co-morbidity presents the exercise professional in cardiac rehabilitation with prescription and programme management challenges that will be further discussed in Chapter 4.

Limitation of functional capacity will often be attributable not to coronary heart disease but to co-morbid conditions. This may mean that functional capacity assessed by means of walking is both ineffective and inappropriate. Can we, therefore, effectively prescribe exercise to accommodate this diversity, and can we implement outcomes to measure the effectiveness of our interventions?

Unfortunately, there does not appear to be a gold standard for measuring physical functioning, either by performance-based or self-report measures (Pepin, *et al.*, 2004), especially in the older patient. As with most aspects of CR it is likely that a variety of measures will need to be considered on an individual patient basis.

In addition, there are proposals of a link between co-morbidity and risk during exercise. Zoghbi, *et al.* (2004) attempted to apply the traditional risk stratification tables of the American Association of Cardiovascular and Pulmonary Rehabilitation (AACVPR, 1999) to a patient population. They also applied a co-morbidity index (CMI) which 'predicts short and long-term mortality rates for a specific medical condition'. This CMI index has been shown to indicate a 'progressive 10-fold increase in mortality as the score increases', with common co-morbid conditions given a weighted score. The researchers concluded that the traditional tool (AACVPR, 1999), but interestingly also the CMI are independent predictors of risk of events during exercise, giving preliminary evidence of a link between co-morbidity and risk during exercise.

However, they also noted that the AACVPR (1999) guidelines were more accurate in predicting high-risk status and events in men, and that the CMI was the significant predictor in women in their study. They suggested that the traditional risk stratification tables may not be sufficient to assess risk across the genders, and that their use should be supplemented with not only risk factor assessment, as proposed in the Canadian (Stone, *et al.*, 2001) tool discussed at the beginning of this chapter, but also with a detailed co-morbidity assessment. They also underline the importance, as did Thow, *et al.* (2003), of staff competency to manage the multitude of non-cardiac co-morbidity among CR participants.

EXERCISE HISTORY

During a holistic assessment of individuals about to embark on CR, exercise history can be an important aspect. It gives the exercise professional a point of reference for the patient's life experience of exercise. The information gained from this subjective discussion can highlight possible barriers to successfully completing a CR, such as having been sedentary and having no exercise history (ACSM, 2001) or having negative memories of physical education at school. This can create a lack of self-efficacy, a known predictor of poor cardiovascular outcomes.

At the other end of the scale, those with a history of competitive sports may highlight a tendency to fail to comply with a given exercise prescription, which itself is recognised as a risk factor for exercise-induced event and therefore a direct link to the risk stratification process. Both the AACPR (1999) and Paul-Labrador, *et al.* (1999) summary of the guidelines describe exceeding exercise prescription as an intermediate risk.

The discussion between CR exercise leader and participant may also highlight cardiac misconceptions, such as a fear of physical exertion, which are generally accepted as related to poorer outcomes and reduced self-efficacy and programme compliance (Maeland and Havik, 1988; SIGN, 2002). The exercise leader can further discuss these misconceptions and attempt to correct them.

PHYSICAL ACTIVITY LEVELS

Cardiac rehabilitation exercise professionals are unlikely to argue with the importance of assessing and documenting baseline physical activity levels or changes in physical activity levels over time. However, despite 40 years of using questionnaires to measure physical activity there are still questions over the best method to achieve it (Shephard, 2003).

There are practical uses of gathering these data:

- as an auditable outcome of physical activity behaviour at key time points, e.g. event/diagnosis, pre- and post-rehabilitation and at one year;

- to educate patients about the definitions and differences between physical activity for general health benefit and exercise for fitness gain and associated benefits (see Chapter 4).

The challenge is to collect meaningful, standardised data. Although many programmes collect a measure of physical activity, there is often wide variation in the tools used, making comparisons between programmes extremely difficult. Self-report measures, although inexpensive and easy to administer (Pepin, *et al.*, 2004), can provide inaccurate information, due to recall bias. Definitions of physical activity, such as those adopted by Health Education Board for Scotland (HEBS) (2001) relate to either moderate or vigorous activity and do not take into account mild activity, such as bowling, slow walking, dancing or golfing, the activities often reported by the CR patient population. A questionnaire being piloted by the British Heart Foundation (BHF), as part of their proposed minimum data set for CR, aims to address this problem (Lewin, *et al.*, 2004).

STAGE OF CHANGE

Assessing a patient's readiness to change in relation to exercise behaviour should always be a component of the exercise professional's assessment. This topic, however, is covered in Chapter 8. An evaluation of a CR programme which forms part of the Scottish Executive Demonstration Project, Have a Heart Paisley (HHP, 2004), reported that individuals assessed to be pre-contemplative and contemplators at baseline were less likely to attend.

Using the stage of change model during assessment can alert the clinician to those individuals least likely to take up or complete CR, enabling them to target resources to those most ready to change. It is also important to ensure that mechanisms are in place for pre-contemplative patients to be referred for other components of rehabilitation, such as smoking cessation, diet and nutrition, psychology and relaxation, and to access exercise services at a later date, should they reach a different stage of physical activity (see Chapter 8 for more on stages of change).

RISK STRATIFICATION FOLLOWING PHASE III

The ultimate aim of CR is the long-term adoption of healthy behaviours by the patient in an attempt to decrease the risk of further events or mortality and to maintain the benefits gained during the rehabilitation programme (SIGN, 2002). The exercise professional must remember that risk stratification is not a static entity. Continuous reassessment and monitoring by the professional and development of self-monitoring skills by the patient are required throughout the course of rehabilitation.

Post-rehabilitation risk stratification should be formally undertaken to:

- ascertain whether the patient is suitable either for discharge to independent exercise or for referral to structured supervised exercise;
- recommend a specific level of supervision, dovetailing with the exercise leader's training and competencies.

As with Phase III cardiac rehabilitation patients, patients moving to phase IV should not be excluded from continuing exercise as far as possible, with decisions based on health screening, risk stratification and also patient preference.

However, as long-term community-based phase IV exercise opportunities are a relatively new development in CR there does not appear to be an extensive body of evidence for risk stratification specifically for post-phase III rehabilitation assessment. It is likely that local programmes have tended to set their own criteria for discharge or referral to phase IV, based on their local patient population, on the availability and type of phase IV opportunities and on the level of qualification of instructors.

The same principles of risk stratification apply as outlined in this chapter; each patient must be considered individually. The ACSM (2001) and the BACR (2002) have published guidelines for independent exercising and referral to phase IV, which is shown in Table 2.4.

Table 2.4. Guidelines for referral to phase IV

Independent exercise with minimal or no supervision (ACSM, 2001)	• Functional capacity ≥8 METs • Cardiac symptoms stable or absent • Appropriate BP response to exercise and recovery • Appropriate ECG response to exercise (i.e. stable/benign arrhythmia, <1 mm ST depression) • Stable heart rate and blood pressure • Safe exercise participation • Knowledge of disease process, own risk factor management and medication use
Transfer to phase IV (BACR, 2002)	• Clinically stable • Able to sustain activities equivalent of 5 METs (i.e. 5 times resting metabolic rate) or at the discretion of phase III personnel • Able to monitor and regulate the intensity of their activity • Able to recognise their optimum level of exercise intensity • Able to acknowledge the importance of and demonstrate a commitment to modifying risk-related behaviour

Many programmes will not have the capacity to continue rehabilitation to individual physical, psychosocial outcomes and individual goals as suggested in Table 2.4. It may be more practical to screen patients prior to discharge using a set of exclusion criteria such as the following, which are currently practiced in the author's programmes.

- SWT <level 7 with cardiac symptoms;
- unable to reach workload of 5 METs/level 7 of SWT with non-cardiac limitation;
- ETT ≤5 METs with cardiac symptoms/2 mm ST depression/silent ischaemia;
- poor LV function (with associated limitation);
- diagnosis of heart failure;
- post-transplant;
- post-ICD insertion;
- refractory angina;
- awaiting CABG;
- awaiting angiogram or PTCA;
- SBP >180 mm hg at rest;
- DBP >100 mm hg at rest.

Phase IV exercise leaders

The BACR (2002) has also, in recent years, established an accredited qualification for community instructors providing exercise to cardiac rehabilitation phase III graduates. This has allowed CR professionals to consider more safely referral for patients who, in the past, would not have had the phase IV option and who would benefit from supervision at that level. There remains a debate as to whether there should be specialist classes for cardiac patients or whether they should be integrated into mainstream exercise classes. Phase III cardiac classes are likely to be male-dominated whereas mainstream community classes are more likely to be female-dominated. Risk stratification should play the pivotal role in the type of class and supervision the exercise professional recommends to each patient, while taking into account their exercise preferences in order to encourage long-term adherence to exercise.

However, even with a trained phase IV exercise leader the patients with complex cardiac histories, complex co-morbidity or high-risk features may require ongoing clinical supervision at a level that is unlikely to be achieved in a community phase IV environment. There is a clear and vital role for the highly skilled exercise professional providing phase III to provide suitable long-term maintenance options for those patients least suited to exercise in the community (Thow, *et al.*, 2003).

PRACTICE ISSUES

Staffing

Although CR is delivered by a multidisciplinary team of health professionals, the exercise component should be delivered by suitably trained exercise professionals, i.e. exercise physiologists, physiotherapists or phase IV BACR exercise professional. Current international guidelines vary in their recommendations for staffing levels, but all agree that the level of staffing required should be driven by the risk stratification of the CR participant within the exercise group. Staff to patient ratio is covered in Chapter 6.

On-site medical supervision

The degree of supervision should be inversely associated with the stability of the CR participant; the higher risk groups require more supervision. Supervised programmes that are equipped with a defibrillator and appropriate emergency drugs will reduce complications. Many studies concur that acute cardiac events can be successfully managed by nursing, AHP and exercise physiologists without medical management (Franklin, *et al.*, 1994; Vongvanich, *et al.*, 1996). Safety issues and emergency procedures are covered in Chapter 6.

Overview

Guidelines for CHD risk stratification were primarily developed to assess prognosis of CHD patients and used to ensure optimal medical management for those individuals. They were adopted by CR programmes as a tool to direct rehabilitation staff to patients who should be offered the exercise component of cardiac rehabilitation and to screen out those who required further interventions, medical or surgical.

Cardiac rehabilitation professionals worldwide have endeavoured to ensure the efficacy and safety of this post-cardiac event intervention including the exercise component. In the adoption of the risk stratification guidelines, as proposed by the foremost authorities, the classification of low to high risk groupings enabled exercise professionals to prescribe safe exercise and to provide adequate monitoring and supervision for each patient in their programmes.

The criteria used to determine the risk classification, first and foremost, examine the medical phenomena associated with subsequent events. Although these are important aspects of the patient assessment, we have demonstrated that the process of risk stratification for the CHD population for exercise cannot be applied in a purely medical manner; by ignoring other factors, i.e.

co-morbidity, smoking, depression, etc., the exercise leader would be under-estimating the risk.

In the past exercise professionals have separated risk classification from risk marker management. Current practice in CR sees the experienced CR leader use a holistic approach to the pre-exercise screening process and, by collating information on a wide range of areas, is able to take account of the numerous factors involved in the complex process of assuring our clients are safely and effectively treated and complete their exercise component of CR.

We suggest that, given the diversity of the client group and the range of personal goals of individual clients, the marrying of risk stratification in the traditional medical sense with the art of the experienced practitioner ensures a safe and effective approach to exercise delivery for this ever-increasing patient group. It will be interesting to monitor whether the UK will adopt the Canadian approach described earlier, which aims to provide a quantifiable indication of overall risk for CHD individuals and mirrors the approach currently used by many experienced practitioners.

In the last 20 years the patient population coming through CR programmes in the UK has changed significantly and there is no doubt that this trend will continue. Although CHD mortality figures are declining, the management of the CHD patient remains a governmental priority. In the years to come, the demographics of the CR population will include many patients we currently consider to be high risk. The implications for future resources of the NHS are considerable. Taking into account the complexity of those most at risk for an exercise-related event, exercise professionals must apply caution in the pre-screening process, if they are to continue to provide safe and effective exercise programmes. CR professionals must not only depend on the traditional risk stratification tools, but must continue to use their clinical reasoning skills and comprehensive assessment to enhance the risk stratification process.

The low-risk patients of today are more often being offered rehabilitation in a community setting. This trend will see our current moderate-risk patients moving to community-based programmes leaving only the high-risk patients to be seen by the CR professional in the hospital setting. This emphasises the importance of training and competence in all the professions delivering this service.

SUMMARY

The concept of a holistic approach to risk stratification is encouraged. This would include the use of traditional medical risk and a broader view of other CHD risk markers and assessment techniques. As there is no gold standard for risk stratification, exercise leaders are encouraged to use those reviewed along with their clinical experience.

REFERENCES

American Association of Cardiovascular and Pulmonary Rehabilitation (AACVPR) (1999) *Guidelines for Cardiac Rehabilitation Programs*, 3rd edn, Human Kinetics, Champaign, IL.

American Association of Cardiovascular and Pulmonary Rehabilitation (AACVPR) (2004) *Guidelines for Cardiac Rehabilitation Programs*, 4th edn, Human Kinetics, Champaign, IL.

American College of Sports Medicine (ACSM) (1995) *Guidelines for Exercise Testing and Prescription*, 5th edn, Williams and Wilkins, London.

American College of Sports Medicine (ACSM) (2001) *ACSM's Resource Manual for Guidelines for Exercise Testing and Prescription*, 4th edn, Williams and Wilkins, London.

American Heart Association (AHA) (2001) Exercise standards: A statement for health care professionals. *Circulation*, **104**, 1694–740.

Armstrong, G., Dunn, M., Bredin, Y., McCuskey, F., Brown, C. (2004) Patients' views on community cardiac rehabilitation. Proceedings of the British Association for Cardiac Rehabilitation Conference.

Association of Chartered Physiotherapists in Cardiac Rehabilitation (ACPICR) (1999) The Chartered Society of Physiotherapy. Standards for the exercise component of Phase III Cardiac Rehabilitation, The Chartered Society of Physiotherapy, London.

Balady, G., Donald, W. (1991) Risk stratification in cardiac rehabilitation. *Journal of Cardiopulmonary Rehabilitation*, **11**, 39–45.

Belardinelli, R. (2003) Arrhythmias during acute and chronic exercise in chronic heart failure. *International Journal of Cardiology*, **90**, 213–18.

British Association for Cardiac Rehabilitation (BACR) (1995) *BACR Guidelines for Cardiac Rehabilitation*, Blackwell Science, Oxford.

British Association for Cardiac Rehabilitation (BACR) (2002) *BACR Exercise Instructor Training Module*, 3rd edn, Human Kinetics, Leeds.

Campeau, L. (1976) Grading of angina pectoris. *Circulation*, **54**, 522.

Castle, A. (2003) Demonstrating critical evaluation skills using Bloom's taxonomy. *International Journal of Therapy and Rehabilitation*, **10**(8), 369–73.

Chang, J., Froelicher, V. (1994) Clinical and exercise test markers of prognosis in patients with stable coronary artery disease. *Current Problems in Cardiology*, **19**, 533–87.

Demers, C., McKelvie, R.S., Nrgassa, A., Yusuf, S. (2001) Reliability, validity, and responsiveness of the six-minute shuttle walk test in patients with heart failure. *American Heart Journal*, **142**, 698–703.

Driving and Vehicle Licensing Agency – At a Glance (DVLA) (2004) Available at http://www.dvla.gov.uk/at_a_glance/ [accessesd 18 Nov 2004].

Fowler, S.J., Singh, S.J., Revill, S. (2005) Reproducibility and validity of the incremental shuttle walking test in patients following coronary artery bypass surgery. *Physiotherapy*, **91**, 22–7.

Franklin, B.A., Blair, S.N., Haskel, W.L., Thompson, P.D., Van Camp, S.P. (1994) Roundtable discussion exercise and cardiac complications: Do the benefits outweigh the risks? *Physician and Sports Medicine*, **22**, 56–68.

Goble, A.J., Worcester, M.U.C. (1999) Best practice guidelines for cardiac rehabilitation and secondary prevention, The Heart Research Centre, Melbourne.

Goebbels, U., Myers, J., Dziekan, G., Muller, P., Kuhn, M., Ratte, R., Dubach, P. (1998) A randomized comparison of exercise training in patients with normal versus reduced ventricular function, *Chest*, **113**(5), 1387–93.

Hachamovitch, R., Berman, D.S., Shaw, J., Kiat, H., Cohen, I., Cabico, J.A. (1998) Incremental prognostic value of myocardial perfusion single photon emission computed tomography for the prediction of cardiac death: Differential stratification for risk of cardiac death and myocardial infarction. *Circulation*, **97**, 535–43.

Have a Heart Paisley: Scottish Demonstration Project for CHD (HHP) (2004) Available at http://www.phis.org.uk/hahp/default.asp [accessed Nov 12 2004].

Health Education Board for Scotland (HEBS) (2001) Summary findings from the 1998 health education population survey. Available at http://www.hebs.scot.nhs.ukresearchcentre/pdf/HEBS98.pdf [accessed Dec 12 2004].

Jesperson, C.M., Hagerup, L., Hollander, N., Launbjerg, J., Linde, N.C., Steinmetz, E. (1993) Exercise-provoked ST segment depression and prognosis in patients recovering from acute myocardial infarction: Significance and pitfalls. *Journal of Internal Medicine*, **233**, 27–32.

Jolliffe, J.A., Rees, K., Taylor, R.S., Thompson, D., Oldridge, N., Ebrahim, S. (2004) Exercise-based rehabilitation for coronary heart disease. Cochrane Database for Systematic Reviews.1. [online] available from http://www.cochrane.org [accessed 14 Feb 2004].

Kavanagh, T., Mertens, D., Hamm, L., Beyene, J., Kennedy, J., Corey, P. (2002) Prediction of long-term prognosis in 12 169 men referred for cardiac rehabilitation. *Circulation*, **106**, 666–71.

Lewin, B. (1997) The psychological and behavioural management of angina. *The Journal of Psychosomatic Research*, **43**(5), 453–62.

Lewin, B., Thompson, D., Roebuck, A. (2004) Development of the BACR/BHF minimum dataset for cardiac rehabilitation. *British Journal of Cardiology*, **11**, 300–1.

Lindsay, G.M. (2004) Risk factor assessment in *Coronary Heart Disease Prevention,* (eds G. Lindsay and A. Gaw), Churchill Livingstone, Edinburgh, pp. 29–52.

Maeland, J., Havik, O. (1988) Self-assessment of health before and after a myocardial infarction. *Social Science Medicine* **27**, 597–605.

McArdle, W.D., Katch, F.I., Katch, V.L. (2001) Exercise physiology; energy, nutrition and human performance, 5th edn, Williams and Wilkins, Baltimore, MD.

McMurray, J.J., Stewart, S. (2000) Epidemiology, aetiology and prognosis of heart failure. *Heart* **83**, 596–602.

Morris, K., Ueshima, K., Kawaguchi, T., Hideg, A., Froelicher, V. (1991) The prognostic value of exercise capacity: a review of the literature. *American Heart Journal*, **122**(5), 1423–31.

Myers, J., Voodi, L., Umann, T., Froelicher, V. (2000) A survey of exercise testing: methods, utilization, interpretation and safety in the VAHCS. *Journal of Cardiopulmonary Rehabilitation*, **20**(4), 251–8.

Myers, J., Prakash, M., Froelicher, V., Do, D., Partington, S., Atwood, E. (2002) Exercise capacity and mortality among men referred for exercise testing. *The New England Journal of Medicine*, **346**(11), 793–801.

New York Heart Association (1994) *Criteria Committee Nomenclature and Criteria for Diagnosis*, 9th edn, Little, Brown, Boston, MA.

O'Connor, G., Buring, J.E., Yusuf, S., Joldhager, S.Z., Olmstead, E.M., Paffenbarger, R.S. (1989) An overview of randomised trials of rehabilitation with exercise after myocardial infarction. *Circulation*, **80**, 234–44.

Oldridge, N., Guyatt, G., Fischer, M.D., Rimm, A.A. (1988) Cardiac rehabilitation after myocardial infarction. *Journal of the American Medical Association*, **260**, 945–50.

Paul-Labrador, M., Vongvanich, P., Merz, C.N.B. (1999) Risk stratification for exercise training in cardiac patients: Do the proposed guidelines work? *Journal of Cardiopulmonary Rehabilitation*, **19**(2), 118–25.

Pepin, V., Alexander, J., Phillips, W. (2004) Physical function assessment in cardiac rehabilitation. *Journal of Cardiopulmonary Rehabilitation*, **24**, 287–95.

Scottish Intercollegiate Guidelines Network (SIGN) (2002) *Cardiac Rehabilitation*, no. 57, Edinburgh.

Shephard, R.J. (2003) Limits to the measurement of habitual physical activity by questionnaires. *British Journal of Sports Medicine*, **37**, 197–206.

Singh, S.J., Morgan, M.C.D.L., Scott, S., Walters, D., Hardman, A.E. (1992) Development of a shuttle-walking test of disability in patients with chronic airways obstruction. *Thorax*, **47**, 1019–24.

Specchia, G., DeServi, S., Scire, A., Assandri, J., Berzuini, C., Angoli, L., *et al.* (1996) Coronary heart disease/atherosclerosis/myocardial infarction: Interaction between exercise training and ejection fraction in predicting prognosis after first myocardial infarction. *Circulation*, **94**(5), 978–82.

Stone, J.A. (ed.) (2005) *Canadian Guidelines for Cardiac Rehabilitation and Cardiovascular Disease Prevention* (2nd edn). Canadian Association of Cardiac Rehabilitation.

Stone, J.A., Cyr, C., Friesen, M., Kennedy-Symonds, H., Stene, R., Smilovitch, M. (2001) On behalf of the Canadian Association for Cardiac Rehabilitation Canadian Guidelines for Cardiac Rehabilitation and atherosclerotic heart disease prevention: A summary. *Canadian Journal Cardiology*, **17**(Suppl B), 3B–30B.

Thow, M., Armstrong, G., Rafferty, D. (2003) Non-cardiac conditions and physiotherapy in phase III cardiac rehabilitation exercise programmes. *Physiotherapy*, **89**(4), 233–7.

Tobin, D., Thow, M.K. (1999) The 10 m shuttle walk test with Holter monitoring: An objective outcome measure for cardiac rehabilitation. *Coronary Health Care*, **3**, 3–17.

Verrill, D., Ashley, R., Witt, K., Forkner, T. (1996) Recommended guidelines for monitoring and supervision of North Carolina phase II/III cardiac rehabilitation programmes: A Position Paper by the North Carolina Cardiopulmonary Rehabilitation Association. *Journal of Cardiopulmonary Rehabilitation*, **16**(1), 9–24.

Vongvanich, P., Paul-Labrador, M.J., Bairey, Merz, C.N. (1996) Safety of medically supervised exercise in a cardiac rehabilitation centre. *American Journal of Cardiology*, **77**, 1383–5.

Zoghbi, G., Sanderson, B., Breland, J., Adams, C., Schumann, C., Bittner, V. (2004) Optimizing risk stratification in cardiac rehabilitation with inclusion of a co-morbidity index. *Journal of Cardiopulmonary Rehabilitation*, **24**, 8–13.

Chapter 3

Exercise Physiology and Monitoring of Exercise in Cardiac Rehabilitation

John Buckley

Chapter outline

The aim of this chapter is to outline the evidence for and the practicalities of safely and effectively using heart rate, ratings of perceived exertion (RPE) and metabolic equivalents (METs) to set and monitor exercise. The chapter will also consider observation as a component of monitoring. The main focus of applying the theory will relate to the intensity monitoring of aerobic exercise, exercise using large muscle groups in a sequential or rhythmical manner.

The exercise leader will make frequent use of all four methods, relative to the prescription of aerobic exercise. Many of these methods are found in nationally and internationally recognised guidelines, including:

- The American Association for Cardiovascular and Pulmonary Rehabilitation (AACVPR, 2004);
- The Scottish Intercollegiate Guidelines Network (SIGN, 2002);
- The American College of Sports Medicine (ACSM, 2000);
- The British Association for Cardiac Rehabilitation (BACR, 1995).

There are benefits and drawbacks (physiologically and psychologically) to the individual use of heart rate, RPE, observation or METs. The approach within this chapter will be first to look at these modalities individually, then to reflect on how the practitioner can integrate their use so that the weaknesses of one may be rectified or 'checked' by one or both of the other three. This integration of modalities forms a brief but very important final section to this chapter.

SAFE AND EFFECTIVE EXERCISE INTENSITY

Exercise *intensity* is felt to be the most important of the four main components of the overload principle of training (McArdle, *et al.*, 2001). The other three components of the overload or dose-response FITT principle are *frequency*, duration (*time*) and mode (*type*) of activity. Hence, the abbreviation FITT is used to describe the 'overload' or 'dose-response' principle. With regard to *exercise intensity* in cardiac patients, the key factors are those that influence:

- The safety of the intensity, to avoid the risk of a clinical cardiovascular event (e.g. ischaemia or arrhythmia) if it were too high, and
- The effectiveness of the programme, determining the intensity threshold or training zone that allows the appropriate physiological adaptations to occur. This would also correspond to the appropriate intensity that allows patients to sustain the required duration of activity for achieving the desired physiological and clinical benefits. If the intensity is too high, patients will not be able to achieve the appropriate duration, and if too low, the full potential of health and clinical benefits from exercise and fitness will not be attained.

There is also the important psychological aspect of determining the correct individualised intensity. Such influences relate to age, gender, mood, self-efficacy and self-esteem (Oldridge and Stoedefalke, 1984; Carlson, *et al.*, 2001; Day, 2003; Yates, *et al.*, 2003). In practical terms this relates to the patients' sense of control or mastery over their exercise, anxieties from the fear of over-exertion causing an event, and attaining enjoyment from the exercise. If the exercise leader fails to achieve these underpinning psychological factors, focusing only on physiological intensity, the required longer-term changes of behaviour for maintaining physical activity at appropriate levels are less likely.

It is important that CR programme teams ensure that patients are confident in working at their physiologically prescribed exercise intensity. This may require the need to build up the patients gradually to their desired intensity over the rehabilitation programme. In order to develop patient self-efficacy for controlling exercise intensity, they should be encouraged to become less reliant on the clinical measures of intensity, such as ECG, heart rate (HR) and METs and to focus, instead, on controlling intensity from their perceptions of exertion that correlate with these clinical measures. A key role of the early phases of CR includes not only enhancing physiological changes but also facilitating patients' learning, identifying and experiencing the correct intensity for attaining and sustaining such changes over the longer term (Song, 2003).

HEART RATE AS A MEASURE

Practicalities of measuring heart rate

If HR is used, it is important that an accurate HR can be measured while the patient is actually exercising. It is the HR while the patient is exercising that provides a marker of both whole body and myocardial strain. The use of a palpated radial pulse requires skill, and for the patient's arm to be very still. Except for static exercise cycling (cycle ergometry), the patient needs to stop the exercise briefly for the pulse to be taken. Even in this very brief period HR drops quickly (De Van, *et al.*, 2004), so that measuring the HR, from the radial pulse, to represent the true exercise intensity is difficult to achieve. The use of a handheld pulse oximeter may help overcome such problems but hand and arm movement still needs to remain relatively still.

Personal HR monitors, with a wireless chest-strap electrode transmitter and wristwatch receiver (e.g. *Polar, Cardiosport* brands), has made a simple, inexpensive and accurate measuring of HR possible. These devices, however, rely on a normal sinus rhythm. If there are disturbances to the normal ECG (e.g. atrial fibrillations or ectopic beats), the monitor will not be able to adjust for these. The next stage up from this is the use of more costly and sophisticated 3-to-12-lead ECG telemetry. For some patients who have undergone coronary bypass surgery, surgical sternal sutures sometimes interfere with the electrodes on the chest strap, and prevent it picking up a valid ECG signal.

As will be discussed in the final section on integrating HR, RPE, observation and METs, many of these limitations can be overcome so as to set exercise intensity safely and effectively for the cardiac patient. A criticism of using equipment to monitor HR is that patients can become over-focused on and obsessive about their HR. There is a good argument for the use of HR monitors for patients who are 'exercise abusers' and require assistance in maintaining a safe intensity.

The physiological rationale for using heart rate

In healthy individuals and cardiac patients, the common aim of using heart rate is to act as a marker of the physiological strain of the exercising skeletal muscles. Specific to the cardiac patient, the role of heart rate (in conjunction with systolic blood pressure) also acts as a key indicator of myocardial strain (Froelicher and Myers, 2000).

As a marker of the body's general physiological strain during aerobic exercise, heart rate is usually described as a percentage of maximal heart rate

(%HRmax). The %HRmax has for many years provided a practical substitute marker of the percentage of maximal aerobic power (%VO₂max). This is based on the assumption that HRmax and VO₂max coincide (Astrand and Rhyming, 1954; Astrand and Christensen, 1964). For an individual, heart rate for a given %VO₂max does not change, regardless of training status, fitness level or age (Skinner, *et al.*, 2003). The use of %HRmax allows for the relative comparison of exercise intensity of people of differing ages. Correspondingly, the use of %VO₂max allows for the relative comparison of individuals of different levels of maximal aerobic power (aerobic fitness). In recognising the heterogeneity of cardiac populations, relative to both age and fitness (Lavie and Milani, 2000), the use of these two relative measures (%HRmax and %VO₂max) allows for the same exercise prescription principles to be applied to all patients.

The %VO₂max, linked to the level of muscle-produced lactate in the blood, is a good indicator of the balance between aerobic and anaerobic metabolic needs of the exercising skeletal muscle (Christensen, 1931; Robinson, 1938; Astrand and Rhyming, 1954; Astrand, *et al.*, 2003). It is such a balance that forms the basis of the intensity targets that are so widely recommended in the recognised guidelines mentioned earlier and to be discussed later in this chapter. The significance of this contribution between aerobic and anaerobic processes (Krogh and Lindhard, 1920) underpins the physiological effectiveness of the exercise session, both in determining the correct intensity and in achieving the required duration of the aerobic exercise session.

A pivotal study by Karvonen, *et al.* (1957) enabled a more accurate coupling between heart rate and %VO₂max. The key aspect was the use of the difference in heart rate between rest and maximal exertion, known as the heart rate reserve. Over a period of training, resting heart rate decreases, whereas maximal heart rate remains much the same; thus, the gap between rest and maximal heart rate increases. This formula accounts for the widening heart rate reserve over the weeks and months of exercise training. The result of this approach is that a given percentage of maximal heart rate reserve (%HRRmax) theoretically represents the same %VO₂max, although a given %HRmax does not represent the same %VO₂max, except near maximal aerobic exercise intensities, as illustrated in Figure 3.1.

More recent recommendations by the ACSM (1998) have referred to a VO₂ reserve method, where there is a matching of heart rate reserve and VO₂ reserve (the difference between resting VO₂ and VO₂max). This method has further increased the accuracy of the link between heart rate and oxygen uptake in representing the work intensity of the exercising skeletal muscle (Swain and Leutholz, 1997). With any of the formulas, accuracy is dependent on the validity of the measured or estimated values. In this case both maximal heart rate and resting heart rate validity need to be considered. Measuring a true resting heart rate requires the patients to monitor themselves at home when they wake first thing in the morning.

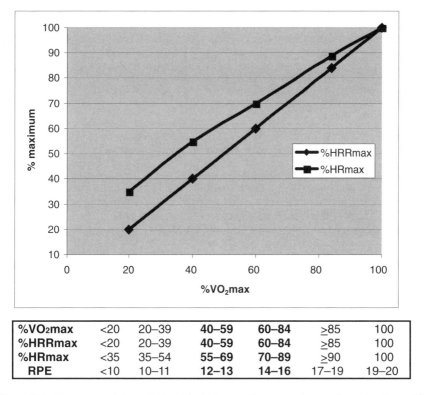

%VO2max	<20	20–39	40–59	60–84	≥85	100
%HRRmax	<20	20–39	40–59	60–84	≥85	100
%HRmax	<35	35–54	55–69	70–89	≥90	100
RPE	<10	10–11	12–13	14–16	17–19	19–20

Figure 3.1. Summary of the relationship between the percentages of maximal aerobic power (%VO2max), maximal heart rate reserve (%HRRmax), maximal heart rate (%HRmax) and Borg's rating of perceived exertion (RPE).
(Adapted from Pollock, *et al.*, 1978; ACSM, 1994, 1998, 2000; Noble and Robertson, 1996.)

MAXIMAL HEART RATE AND PEAK HEART RATE

Since the 1930s, the maximal heart rate of an individual has been shown to approximate a value equal to subtracting one's age from 220 beats per minute (beats·min^{-1}) (Christensen, 1931; Robinson, 1938; Astrand and Rhyming in Astrand, *et al.*, 2003). More recently, Tanaka, *et al.*, (2001) reported that 220 minus age underestimated maximal heart rate in older adults, which would be relevant to cardiac populations. Nevertheless, with age as the main predictor of maximal heart rate in all the above studies, this does not filter out the more individualised factors of autonomic regulation that influence heart rate from rest up to maximal exertion. Astrand and Christensen (1964) and Astrand, *et al.* (1973) cautioned that the error around the prediction of maximal heart rate based on age had a standard deviation of +/– 10 beats·min^{-1}. This means that

Heart rate (HR) and ejection fraction (EF) response curves

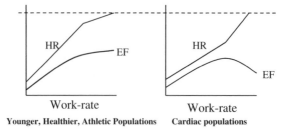

Younger, Healthier, Athletic Populations   **Cardiac populations**

Figure 3.2. Myocardial performance to increase exercise intensities.
The left panel demonstrates that in the healthy individual ejection fraction plateaus at
50–60% of VO_2max and the increase in heart rate has a turn-point in the region of
60–80% VO_2max before it reaches maximal levels (dotted line). This turn point has
been hypothesised to be associated with the lactate threshold.

The right panel shows that at similar relative intensities, myocardial performance
begins to deteriorate in cardiac populations, where there is a loss of stroke volume
associated with a decreased ejection fraction; heart rate rises in an accelerating fashion
in an attempt to compensate and to preserve cardiac output.

(Adapted from Conconi, *et al.*, 1982 and Pokan, *et al.*, 1998.)

in some individuals their actual maximal heart rate could be as much as 20
beats·min^{-1} above or below the age-estimated maximum. For a healthy individual an error in over-prescribing a target heart rate would result in the discomfort of overexertion. However, for the cardiac patient such an error could
be enough to trigger an event of ischaemia, an arrhythmia or a failure of
cardiac output to match the systemic circulatory demands of vigorous
exercise (Figure 3.2).

It is likely, however, that such individuals will have been through an appropriate ETT (exercise tolerance test), which is assumed to provide a safe upper
heart rate limit. It is important to acknowledge that even when an ETT is
carried out it is possible that neither a true maximal heart rate will have been
attained nor a conclusive intensity identified where a clinical cardiac change
occurred. The typical clinical changes include ST-segment displacement
(e.g. ST-segment depression suggestive of ischaemia), onset of arrhythmias or
tachycardias, or a failure of increases in cardiac output to match increases in
exercise intensity (recognised via blood pressure monitoring) (ACSM, 2000).

If an individual completes an ETT without any key clinical events, the
highest heart rate attained may need to be described as a 'peak heart rate'.
This is because in many cases the criteria for a true maximal test have not been
met (ACSM, 2000). Many ETTs are stopped when the patient attains their
age-estimated maximal heart rate. If the patient is clearly not at a point of volitional fatigue, their true maximal heart rate will actually be above this level.
Subsequent exercise programming based on the heart rate at test termination

could be under-prescribed in terms of intensity. This does, however, leave a margin of safety. In this case it is better to describe the prescribed intensity in relation to a peak heart rate (HRpeak). The same holds true when using the Karvonen (1957) heart rate reserve formula. If all exercise leaders on the rehabilitation team have a clear understanding of the differences between HRmax and HRpeak, then it will be clear whether the patient is exercising relative to their maximal capacity or a level which was determined relative to a clinical event or some other limiting factor (e.g. musculoskeletal problems) highlighted during the test. If, on the other hand, a patient stops due to true volitional fatigue, then whatever heart rate they were at (regardless of it being less than 220 minus age) would be a true maximum. This is often the case when the patient being tested is on beta-blocking medication and completes the test without any clinical events, representing a true beta-blocked maximal heart rate.

Tests may be terminated inconclusively, when neither a maximum heart rate nor a heart rate corresponding to a clinical event is determined. This leaves the exercise leader with limited knowledge of what constitutes a safe training heart rate. This problem often relates to factors influenced by the testing protocol or mode of testing (e.g. treadmill) (Myers and Froelicher, 1993). Such factors include changes in the speed and/or gradient of the treadmill, which are too much for the patient who is either limited by neuro-musculoskeletal mobility problems, pulmonary pathology, circulatory pathology (e.g. peripheral vascular disease) or fear and anxiety. The exercise leader often has to use a process of trial and error, or rely on RPE to determine an appropriate intensity based on patient comments, symptoms and visual observation. This may be the only possible option, but it needs to consider two issues:

- The patient may suffer from silent ischaemia, exercise-induced arrhythmias or failure to increase cardiac output at heart rates that could have occurred at levels not much above where the test was prematurely terminated;
- The patient's progress may be hindered (physiologically and psychologically), due to the clinicians taking a more cautious approach.

With regard to patients having undergone percutaneous coronary interventions (PCI) or revascularisation procedures (coronary angioplasty, stenting or bypass graft surgery), it is uncommon in the UK for these patients subsequently to have an exercise ETT. These patients (especially PCI) may, however, have been through an exercise test recently, prior to their revascularisation and hence these data (if recent) will still have some valuable information reflecting functional capacity for exercise intensity prescription purposes. Communication with the relevant physician or surgeon is required to qualify the success of the procedure in terms of rectification of exertion-related ischaemia, arrhythmias or myocardial performance. In the absence of an exercise ETT, sub-maximal tests can be used to assess functional capacity and subsequently set target intensity, including heart rate. Such tests are limited as a valid means for risk stratification, diagnosis or prognosis. If a PCI or revascularised patient does develop symptoms over time associated with ischaemia, arrhythmias or myocardial dysfunction, an exercise stress test and other related tests are advisable.

HEART RATE TARGET ZONES

Having a close estimate, or better still an actual maximal heart rate, will greatly increase the accuracy and appropriateness of the exercise intensity being prescribed. However, as described above, in many cases a true maximal heart rate will not be available. This next section focuses more closely on the setting of target zones or exercise heart rates (Table 3.1) in light of two aspects:

1. The safety threshold for preventing myocardial complications on exertion;
2. The effective threshold for attaining beneficial physiological adaptations, which is linked to the patient's training status. The training status influences the heart rate relationship with both $\%VO_2max$ and the 'lactate threshold'.

THE SAFE HEART RATE

Before considering the target heart rate from a physiological training perspective, the safe exercise HR has to be regarded as the prime governor to the upper limit of exercise (Coplan, *et al.*, 1986). This specifically refers to the heart rate at which medically significant myocardial events can occur (e.g. ischaemia, arrhythmia and failure to increase cardiac output). Such a level can only be determined from a standard ETT. Based on evidence for individuals with silent myocardial ischaemia (Hoberg, *et al.*, 1990) the ACSM (2000) recommend that

Table 3.1. Recommended aerobic exercise intensities relative to the percentage of maximal oxygen uptake ($\%VO_2max$), maximal heart rate reserve ($\%HRRmax$) and maximal heart rate ($\%HRmax$)

Guideline	ACSM (1994, 2000)	BACR (1995), SIGN (2002)
$\%VO_2max*$	40%–85%	40%–60%**
$\%HRRmax$	40%–85%	40%–60%**
$\%HRmax$	55%–90%	60%–75%**

*The term VO_2max is used in this case for reasons of simplicity but it must be noted that guidelines vary in the use of VO_2peak or maximal $VO_2reserve$.
**In Britain the upper intensity limit is lower than that for the USA because British programmes do not typically use sophisticated ECG heart rate monitoring during the actual exercise sessions, except in cases of higher risk patients.

the upper HR limit should be set at least 10 beats·min^{-1} below the level associated with myocardial dysfunction. In patients who do get typical symptoms that relate to ischaemia or cardiac output dysfunction (angina and breathlessness, respectively), it is possible that these symptoms could arise at a point higher than the actual onset of the clinically measured significant change. Hence, it would be unwise to use these symptoms as a reference point for determining the upper HR training limit. It is therefore important first to acknowledge the safe heart rate limit, relative to the effective physiological training HR limits, as outlined in Table 3.1.

The beneficial target heart rate

Beneficial HR target selection and progression assumes that the patient has developed the skill and confidence to exercise at these recommended intensities. The target range for the recommended physiologically effective heart rate, as summarised in Table 3.1, is directly linked with the training status of the individual. The more training an individual has done, from the perspective of frequency (times per week) and longevity (>4 weeks), the greater the percentage of maximum (HR, HRR or VO_2) at which that individual will need to work in order to gain further benefits (Ekblom, *et al.*, 1968). This leads to the concept of considering intensity progression relative to both work rate and heart rate.

Progression of exercise intensity and heart rate

This section provides the rationale for using the recommended target heart rates summarised in Table 3.1 as a range of values. The sedentary patient is thus prescribed exercise starting at the low end of the recommended heart rate range. Over the course of the first three to six months of exercise the patient should progress the intensity to elicit heart rates in the middle of the range. In the longer term, if the patient continues to exercise regularly, they could progress to the higher end of the target heart rate zone. All of this assumes that these targets are 10 beats·min^{-1} below the clinically significant heart rate as described in the section on the safe heart rate. The need for later progressions in exercise intensity provides an important rationale for having qualified exercise advisors available to patients in phase IV CR. This type of exercise leader is available to discuss with the patient appropriate changes to their exercise regime in the longer term.

Exercise leaders should be aware that target heart rates can be adjusted in the future. The heart rate intensity can be used to increase the training effect. For some patients the duration may be used as the variable. It is not incorrect to assume that the progression of intensity will automatically occur if the patient exercises to the same given heart rate; the work rate for a given heart rate will increase as fitness improves. However, this assumption only reflects one of the two main training adaptations to regular aerobic exercise: an increase in VO_2max. The other physiological adaptation, as shown clearly in three studies involving cardiac patients, is that with training, individuals can sustain exercise at a higher proportion (percentage) of their VO_2max (Sullivan, *et al.*, 1989; Meyer, *et al.*, 1990; Goodman, *et al.*, 1999). In these three studies, this phenomenon was closely allied to the amount of lactic acid produced at a given VO_2, a phenomenon which has been known for many years (Edwards, *et al.*, 1939; Ekblom, *et al.*, 1968). The importance of this is that improvements in aerobic power (VO_2max) and endurance capacity (the intensity at the lactate threshold) in cardiac patients, compared to healthy individuals, is mostly due to the adaptations of skeletal muscle and not of the myocardium (Hiatt, 1991). Because the key agent in increasing VO_2max in cardiac patients is skeletal muscle, it is important to ensure that this tissue is challenged as effectively as possible. This is even more apparent in the training adaptations of the older or heart failure patient (Sullivan, *et al.*, 1989; Ades, *et al.*, 1996).

HEART RATE, MYOCARDIAL STRAIN AND PERFORMANCE

There is a direct link between HR and myocardial strain, performance and dysfunction. However, the contractility of the myocardium is also a function of the stroke volume that results from the heart wall tension produced during diastole and the force of contraction during systole. This, together with the rate of contraction, produces a given cardiac output. It is both the rate and force of contraction of the myocardium that determine the oxygen demand or uptake (MVO_2) of the heart (Froelicher and Myers, 2000). Hence, the performance of the ventricles is determined by the amount of pressure that can or needs to be created during systole. The systolic pressure therefore provides an indirect means of indicating the force of contraction. A practical index of myocardial strain has thus been described as the product of HR and systolic blood pressure and given the single term rate pressure product (RPP) or double pressure product (Gobel, *et al.*, 1978). In this study, the use of systolic blood pressure in conjunction with HR provided a better index of MVO_2 than HR alone.

From a practical perspective, the concept of MVO_2 and rate pressure product is best highlighted when comparing upper body and lower body exercise. Miles, *et al.* (1989) demonstrated in healthy individuals and cardiac patients that for the same oxygen uptake, blood pressure is higher for upper body compared to lower body exercise. This is due to the smaller vascular bed in the arms, compared to the legs, and the added isometric contractions in the thoracic region to provide a stabilising base for the shoulder joints and muscles. Therefore, if an individual exercises at his or her set target HR with the upper body, rather than with the lower body, the result will be a higher systolic pressure, giving rise to a greater rate pressure product or MVO_2.

For example, if a patient's target HR is 120 beats·min^{-1}, and during lower body exercise their systolic blood pressure is 150 mmHg, then the rate pressure product will equal 18 000 (120 × 150). Knowing that upper body exercise will have a greater systolic blood pressure (perhaps 165 mmHg), then at the same target HR of 120 beats·min^{-1} the rate pressure product would be 19 800 (120 × 165). This represents a 10% increase in myocardial oxygen demand, which is equivalent to raising a person's HR by 7 to 10 beats·min^{-1} during lower body exercise, such as walking or cycling.

This example shows that it would be wise to reduce the target HR by 5-to-10 beats·min^{-1} during activities involving the arms. Furthermore, this may also prevent unnecessary muscular fatigue, as it has been shown that, for a variety of reasons, both healthy individuals and cardiac patients are metabolically less efficient during activities that involve the arms compared with the legs (Secher, 1993; Kang, *et al.*, 1997; Buckley, *et al.*, 1999a).

OTHER CONSIDERATIONS FOR HEART RATE MONITORING ASSOCIATED WITH CHANGES IN MYOCARDIAL PERFORMANCE

Figure 3.2 (see page 52) illustrates the optimisation of myocardial perform- ance by the interaction between HR and ejection fraction, which is directly related to stroke volume (Conconi, *et al.*, 1982; Pokan, *et al.*, 1998). For the healthy individual, although stroke volume reaches a maximum at about 50 to 60% of VO_2max, myocardial performance is preserved as HR continues to rise towards maximal levels. In cardiac patients, the right-hand panel of Figure 3.2 demonstrates a deterioration of ejection fraction as HR progresses towards maximum. In an attempt to preserve cardiac output, HR rises in an acceler- ating manner, which further decreases diastole and thus myocardial perfusion time. The risk of ischaemia is heightened and/or blood pressure does not rise to meet the circulation required for the aerobic demands of the muscles. Not only does the HR rate shorten diastole that can affect myocardial perfu- sion, but it can also reduce ventricular filling (Poulsen, 2001). Reduced ven- tricular filling leads to reduced stroke volume by way of the Frank-Starling mechanism, and hence myocardial performance may not match the circula- tory needs of the exercise being performed. The change in rate pressure product has also been demonstrated to behave similarly to ejection fraction (as seen in Figure 3.2), where it begins to decrease at higher heart rates (Omiya, *et al.*, 2004).

The rate pressure product turn point identified by Omiya, *et al.* (2004) is also correlated with both the ventilatory and lactate thresholds (the upper limit recommended for continuous aerobic exercise at which a training benefit is optimised). This finding corresponds with the original concept of the heart rate turn-point reported by Conconi, *et al.* (1982) (Figure 3.2). However, some debate exists over its merits as a means of estimating the lactate threshold because the relationship may be strongly dependent on the exercise testing protocol used (Bodner and Rhodes, 2000). Nevertheless, from a myocardial perspective, there is no doubt in all these reports that at higher intensities, HR does not continue to rise in a linear fashion, which provides the evidence of a decreased myocardial performance. For the practitioner this means that encouraging patients to work at high HR is not prudent in the early stages of CR. Although Ehsani, *et al.* (1982) did show that myocardial contractile improvements could occur from exercising at higher exercise intensities, this was with three to four days of training over a 12-month period. For a few cardiac patients, over many years of progressive overload aerobic training, higher heart rates can be attained and are safe (Thow, *et al.*, 2004). Few studies have evaluated the physiological outcomes after years of CR exercise.

THE PRACTICALITIES OF SETTING TARGET HEART RATES

From ETT results, the HRpeak can be used in either the %HRpeak or %HRRpeak (Karvonen HR reserve method) formulas. If a true maximal HR has been attained, then the annotation would be %HRmax or %HRRmax, respectively. When using the age-estimated maximal HR formula of 220 minus age (years) or the formula recommended by Tanaka, *et al.* (2001) of 208 minus (age years × 0.7), then the convention is to use %HRmax.

Table 3.2 provides a quick calculation for determining a target heart rate for a given %HRmax or %HRpeak, determined either from an age-estimation or an exercise test, respectively. Table 3.3 does the same, but for a patient on beta-blocking medication, where sub-maximal and peak exercising HR is reduced by between 20 and 40 beats per minute (Davies and Sargeant, 1979; Eston and Connelly, 1996; Liu, *et al.*, 2000).

The Karovonen heart rate reserve method for determining a target HR, which can be used from either an exercise test peak HR (HRpeak), a maximal HR (HRmax), or from the age estimated HRmax formulas above, is as follows:

Target heart rate = %target × (HRpeak/max − HRrest) + HRrest
%target = the desired percentage (e.g. 65%) of maximum at which the patient will exercise
HRrest = the patient's resting heart rate

Table 3.4 provides a quick calculation of the %HRmax or peak.

Table 3.2. Target heart rate determination

	For %HRmax calculation from age-estimated maximum (220 − age) or from %HRpeak taken from an exercise test														
Age (years)	15	20	25	30	35	40	45	50	55	60	65	70	75	80	85
HRpeak	205	200	195	190	185	180	175	170	165	160	155	150	145	140	135
Heart rate (bpm)															
40	20%	20%	21%	21%	22%	22%	23%	24%	24%	25%	26%	27%	28%	29%	30%
45	20%	23%	23%	24%	24%	25%	26%	26%	27%	28%	29%	30%	31%	32%	33%
50	23%	25%	26%	26%	27%	28%	29%	29%	30%	31%	32%	33%	34%	36%	37%
55	25%	28%	28%	29%	30%	31%	31%	32%	33%	34%	35%	37%	38%	39%	41%
60	27%	30%	31%	32%	32%	33%	34%	35%	36%	38%	39%	40%	41%	43%	44%
65	30%	33%	33%	34%	35%	36%	37%	38%	39%	41%	42%	43%	45%	46%	48%
70	32%	35%	36%	37%	38%	39%	40%	41%	42%	44%	45%	47%	48%	50%	52%
75	34%	38%	38%	39%	41%	42%	43%	44%	45%	47%	48%	50%	52%	54%	56%
80	36%	40%	41%	42%	43%	44%	46%	47%	48%	50%	52%	53%	55%	57%	59%
85	39%	43%	44%	45%	46%	47%	49%	50%	52%	53%	55%	57%	59%	61%	63%
90	41%	45%	46%	47%	49%	50%	51%	53%	55%	56%	58%	60%	62%	64%	67%
95	43%	48%	49%	50%	51%	53%	54%	56%	58%	59%	61%	63%	66%	68%	70%
100	46%	50%	51%	53%	54%	56%	57%	59%	61%	63%	65%	67%	69%	71%	74%
105	48%	53%	54%	55%	57%	58%	60%	62%	64%	66%	68%	70%	72%	75%	78%
110	50%	55%	56%	58%	59%	61%	63%	65%	67%	69%	71%	73%	76%	79%	81%
115	52%	58%	59%	61%	62%	64%	66%	68%	70%	72%	74%	77%	79%	82%	85%
120	55%	60%	62%	63%	65%	67%	69%	71%	73%	75%	77%	80%	83%	86%	89%
125	57%	63%	64%	66%	68%	69%	71%	74%	76%	78%	81%	83%	86%	89%	93%
130	59%	65%	67%	68%	70%	72%	74%	76%	79%	81%	84%	87%	90%	93%	96%
135	62%	68%	69%	71%	73%	75%	77%	79%	82%	84%	87%	90%	93%	96%	100%

Table 3.2. *Continued*

For %HRmax calculation from age-estimated maximum (220 – age) or from %HRpeak taken from an exercise test

Age (years)	15	20	25	30	35	40	45	50	55	60	65	70	75	80	85
HRpeak	205	200	195	190	185	180	175	170	165	160	155	150	145	140	135
140	64%	70%	72%	74%	76%	78%	80%	82%	85%	88%	90%	93%	97%	100%	
145	66%	73%	74%	76%	78%	81%	83%	85%	88%	91%	94%	97%	100%		
150	68%	75%	77%	79%	81%	83%	86%	88%	91%	94%	97%	100%			
155	71%	78%	79%	82%	84%	86%	89%	91%	94%	97%	100%				
160	73%	80%	82%	84%	86%	89%	91%	94%	97%	100%					
165	75%	83%	85%	87%	89%	92%	94%	97%	100%						
170	78%	85%	87%	89%	92%	94%	97%	100%							
175	80%	88%	90%	92%	95%	97%	100%								
180	82%	90%	92%	95%	97%	100%									
185	84%	93%	95%	97%	100%										
190	87%	95%	97%	100%											
195	89%	98%	100%												
200	91%	100%													

To determine the target heart rate, find either the patient's maximal heart rate based on age or the true maximum of peak determined from an exercise test along the top row. Read down the column below this figure to the desired relative intensity, expressed as a percentage of maximal or peak. Then read back across that row to the left hand column, which provides the target heart rate in beats·min⁻¹.

Adapted from Christensen, 1931; Robinson, 1938; and Astrand and Rhyming, 1954; cited in Astrand, *et al.*, 2003.

Table 3.3. Beta-blocked target heart rate determination

	For %HRmax calculation from age-estimated maximum (220 – age) or from %HRpeak taken from an exercise test														
Age (years)	15	20	25	30	35	40	45	50	55	60	65	70	75	80	85
HRpeak	175	170	165	160	155	150	145	140	135	130	125	120	115	110	105
Target Heart rate (bpm)															
40	23%	24%	24%	25%	26%	27%	28%	29%	30%	31%	32%	33%	35%	36%	38%
45	26%	26%	27%	28%	29%	30%	31%	32%	33%	35%	36%	38%	39%	41%	43%
50	29%	29%	30%	31%	32%	33%	34%	36%	37%	38%	40%	42%	43%	45%	48%
55	31%	32%	33%	34%	35%	37%	38%	39%	41%	42%	44%	46%	48%	50%	52%
60	34%	35%	36%	38%	39%	40%	41%	43%	44%	46%	48%	50%	52%	55%	57%
65	37%	38%	39%	41%	42%	43%	45%	46%	48%	50%	52%	54%	57%	59%	62%
70	40%	41%	42%	44%	45%	47%	48%	50%	52%	54%	56%	58%	61%	64%	67%
75	43%	44%	45%	47%	48%	50%	52%	54%	56%	58%	60%	63%	65%	68%	71%
80	46%	47%	48%	50%	52%	53%	55%	57%	59%	62%	64%	67%	70%	73%	76%
85	49%	50%	52%	53%	55%	57%	59%	61%	63%	65%	68%	71%	74%	77%	81%
90	51%	53%	55%	56%	58%	60%	62%	64%	67%	69%	72%	75%	78%	82%	86%
95	54%	56%	58%	59%	61%	63%	66%	68%	70%	73%	76%	79%	83%	86%	90%
100	57%	59%	61%	63%	65%	67%	69%	71%	74%	77%	80%	83%	87%	91%	95%
105	60%	62%	64%	66%	68%	70%	72%	75%	78%	81%	84%	88%	91%	95%	100%
110	63%	65%	67%	69%	71%	73%	76%	79%	81%	85%	88%	92%	96%	100%	
115	66%	68%	70%	72%	74%	77%	79%	82%	85%	88%	92%	96%	100%		
120	69%	71%	73%	75%	77%	80%	83%	86%	89%	92%	96%	100%			

Table 3.3. *Continued*

Age (years)	15	20	25	30	35	40	45	50	55	60	65	70	75	80	85
HRpeak	175	170	165	160	155	150	145	140	135	130	125	120	115	110	105
125	71%	74%	76%	78%	81%	83%	86%	89%	93%	96%	100%				
130	74%	76%	79%	81%	84%	87%	90%	93%	96%	100%					
135	77%	79%	82%	84%	87%	90%	93%	96%	100%						
140	80%	82%	85%	88%	90%	93%	97%	100%							
145	83%	85%	88%	91%	94%	97%	100%								
150	86%	88%	91%	94%	97%	100%									
155	89%	91%	94%	97%	100%										
160	91%	94%	97%	100%											
165	94%	97%	100%												
170	97%	100%													
175	100%														
180															
185															
190															

For %HRmax calculation from age-estimated maximum (220 – age) or from %HRpeak taken from an exercise test

To determine the target heart rate, find either the patient's maximal heart rate based on age or the true maximum of peak determined from an exercise test along the top row. Read down the column below this figure to the desired relative intensity, expressed as a percentage of maximal or peak. Then read back across that row to the left hand column, which provides the target heart rate in beats·min⁻¹.
Adapted from Davies and Sargeant 1979; Eston and Connelly, 1996, Liu, *et al.*, 2000.

Table 3.4. Calculation tables of 50% to 70% of maximal or peak heart rate reserve

50%HRR max/peak	HR rest 45	HR rest 50	HR rest 55	HR rest 60	HR rest 65	HR rest 70	HR rest 75	HR rest 80	HR rest 85	HR rest 90	HR rest 95
HR max/pk											
185	115	118	120	123	125	128	130	133	135	138	140
180	113	115	118	120	123	125	128	130	133	135	138
175	110	113	115	118	120	123	125	128	130	133	135
170	108	110	113	115	118	120	123	125	128	130	133
165	105	108	110	113	115	118	120	123	125	128	130
160	103	105	108	110	113	115	118	120	123	125	128
155	100	103	105	108	110	113	115	118	120	123	125
150	98	100	103	105	108	110	113	115	118	120	123
145	95	98	100	103	105	108	110	113	115	118	120
140	93	95	98	100	103	105	108	110	113	115	118
135	90	93	95	98	100	103	105	108	110	113	115
130	88	90	93	95	98	100	103	105	108	110	113
125	85	88	90	93	95	98	100	103	105	108	110
120	83	85	88	90	93	95	98	100	103	105	108
115	80	83	85	88	90	93	95	98	100	103	105
110	78	80	83	85	88	90	93	95	98	100	103
105	75	78	80	83	85	88	90	93	95	98	100
100	73	75	78	80	83	85	88	90	93	95	98

Table 3.4. *Continued*

65%HRR max/peak	HR rest 45	HR rest 50	HR rest 55	HR rest 60	HR rest 65	HR rest 70	HR rest 75	HR rest 80	HR rest 85	HR rest 90	HR rest 95
HR max/pk											
185	136	138	140	141	143	145	147	148	150	152	154
180	133	135	136	138	140	142	143	145	147	149	150
175	130	131	133	135	137	138	140	142	144	145	147
170	126	128	130	132	133	135	137	139	140	142	144
165	123	125	127	128	130	132	134	135	137	139	141
160	120	122	123	125	127	129	130	132	134	136	137
165	123	125	127	128	130	132	134	135	137	139	141
160	120	122	123	125	127	129	130	132	134	136	137
155	117	118	120	122	124	125	127	129	131	132	134
150	113	115	117	119	120	122	124	126	127	129	131
145	110	112	114	115	117	119	121	122	124	126	128
140	107	109	110	112	114	116	117	119	121	123	124
135	104	105	107	109	111	112	114	116	118	119	121
130	100	102	104	106	107	109	111	113	114	116	118
125	97	99	101	102	104	106	108	109	111	113	115
120	94	96	97	99	101	103	104	106	108	110	111
115	91	92	94	96	98	99	101	103	105	106	108
110	87	89	91	93	94	96	98	100	101	103	105
105	84	86	88	89	91	93	95	96	98	100	102
100	81	83	84	86	88	90	91	93	95	97	98

70%HRR max/peak	45	50	55	60	65	70	75	80	85	90	95
HR max/pk											
185	143	145	146	148	149	151	152	154	155	157	158
180	140	141	143	144	146	147	149	150	152	153	155
175	136	138	139	141	142	144	145	147	148	150	151
170	133	134	136	137	139	140	142	143	145	146	148
165	129	131	132	134	135	137	138	140	141	143	144
160	126	127	129	130	132	133	135	136	138	139	141
165	129	131	132	134	135	137	138	140	141	143	144
160	126	127	129	130	132	133	135	136	138	139	141
155	122	124	125	127	128	130	131	133	134	136	137
150	119	120	122	123	125	126	128	129	131	132	134
145	115	117	118	120	121	123	124	126	127	129	130
140	112	113	115	116	118	119	121	122	124	125	127
135	108	110	111	113	114	116	117	119	120	122	123
130	105	106	108	109	111	112	114	115	117	118	120
125	101	103	104	106	107	109	110	112	113	115	116
120	98	99	101	102	104	105	107	108	110	111	113
115	94	96	97	99	100	102	103	105	106	108	109
110	91	92	94	95	97	98	100	101	103	104	106
105	87	89	90	92	93	95	96	98	99	101	102
100	84	85	87	88	90	91	93	94	96	97	99

Choose the table that is for a target of 50%, 65% or 70% of maximal heart rate reserve. Read down the left hand column to the patient's maximal heart rate or peak heart rate determined from an age estimated maximum or an exercise test, respectively. Then read across the row that corresponds to the patient's resting heart rate, noted at the top of the column.
Adapted from Karvonen, *et al.*, 1957.

TARGET HEART RATE RESPONSE NUANCES DURING THE EXERCISE SESSION

Two factors can alter the theoretical relationship between exercise work rate and HR during an exercise session:

1. Cardiovascular drift;
2. Exercises performed using an interval approach, where each station or interval of exercise lasts less than two minutes.

Cardiovascular drift

The basic premise of cardiovascular drift is that after 10 minutes of exercise, HR will rise in spite of no change in the work rate or oxygen cost of the exercise being performed (Coyle and Gonzales-Alonso, 2001). There are a number of factors, which continue to be debated, in this effect (Ajisaka, *et al.*, 2000; Cheatham, *et al.*, 2000; Coyle and Gonzales-Alonso, 2001). The agreed fact is that, for a given oxygen uptake, cardiac output must remain constant. What is still debatable is the cause of cardiovascular drift including:

- a decrease in peripheral vascular resistance that leads to a drop in blood pressure as a result of an increase in skin blood flow to meet the needs of thermo-regulation, in light of the fact that blood pressure is a function of the stroke volume component of cardiac output and total peripheral resistance;
- a decrease in plasma volume, due to either dehydration or a shift of fluid from the vascular to the interstitial tissues of the exercising muscle;
- a drop in stroke volume, either as a function of one or both of the factors above, where venous return has decreased and impairs the Frank-Starling mechanism, or possibly, and more simply that a raised HR reduces the time for ventricular filling.

From the exercise leader's perspective, the one undeniable point is that over the duration of an exercise rehabilitation session the target HR should allow for an upward drift in HR by as much as 10 beats·min^{-1}.

Heart rate response during interval-type exercise

Interval circuit exercise is specifically beneficial to individuals with low functional capacity, left ventricular dysfunction or concomitant pulmonary or peripheral circulatory disease exercise limitations (Cachovan, *et al.*, 1976; Maass, *et al.*, 1983; Meyer, *et al.*, 1990; Cooper, 2001).

The use of interval circuit exercise is a typical feature in the UK for phase III and IV rehabilitation programmes. Interval training permits the patient to produce a greater amount of work in a training session if the training periods are spaced between periods of lower intensity work. These lower intensity bouts, called active recovery (AR) periods, are between 30 seconds and 1 minute in duration. A deconditioned patient may only be able to maintain a training intensity exercise for a few minutes before becoming too fatigued to continue.

Other practical reasons for using the interval circuit format include the lack of specialist exercise facilities, where rehabilitation gymnasia are multipurpose, and the area needs to be set up and cleared for a variety of uses. This is addressed by the characteristics of interval training which allows for the use of very basic exercise equipment (hand weights, steps, shuttle walks, callisthenic-type movements, etc.) and typically results in an interval approach where patients exercise for no more than three minutes at each station. The total duration of exercise, however, is aimed at accumulating the recommended minimum of at least 20 minutes of aerobic activity (ACSM, 2000). The AR intervals are typically no more than one minute. The progression is to gradually remove the active-rest intervals towards achieving at least 20 minutes of continuous activity.

For patients using interval circuit training, the differences in HR response compared to continuous activity need to be acknowledged. It has long been known that it takes at least two minutes for HR to rise and level off, following the initiation of constant sub-maximal exercise workload (Saltin, *et al.*, 2000). This time lag is a function of the response time of the sympathetic neuro-humoral regulation of HR, relative to the required systemic circulatory and metabolic demands. Because interval training often has exercise stations lasting less than two minutes, the theoretical matching of HR to muscular work output will not occur. If patients are attaining their aerobic target HR in this short period (<2 mins) they will actually be working at an intensity that would elicit an HR above their target, if the activity were sustained continuously (>2 mins).

Inadvertently, this is beneficial, because it is metabolically challenging to the skeletal muscle. In addition, there is a built-in safety margin for the HR. Before HR begins to approach its critical level, the patient starts to decrease intensity as part of AR. However, over the course of a rehabilitation session, there is cardiovascular drift and an increased likelihood of muscular fatigue. This latter point could cause a potential loss of sense of achievement for the patient if the intensity is too high. With too high an intensity, the accumulation of lactic acid will prolong both metabolic recovery and heart rate recovery (McArdle, *et al.*, 2001). This is due to both the raised aerobic metabolism needed to clear the lactate from the system and lactate's sympathetic nervous system stimulating properties. The concept of the cool-down is discussed in more depth in Chapter 5 on programme design.

Figure 3.3 provides an example of the differences in an individual's HR at the same treadmill speeds during one-minute, compared to three-minute stages. In this individual, when the intensity requires greater than 60% HRmax

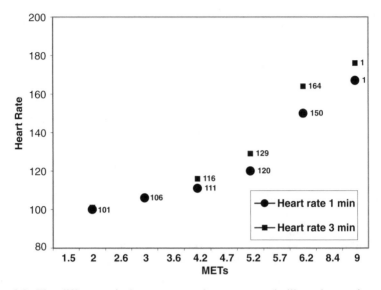

Figure 3.3. The difference in heart rate at the same treadmill work rate (metabolic equivalents; METs) on two separate tests; one test where the duration at each stage was one minute and the other for three minutes at each stage.

(JP Buckley (unpublished) 2004, Exercise Laboratory, School of Health and Rehabilitation, Keele University, UK.)

(120 beats·min^{-1}), the difference in HR by prolonging exercise at a given work rate from one minute to three minutes is as much as 10 beats·min^{-1}.

RATINGS OF PERCEIVED EXERTION

How the patients develop the ability to perceive how hard they are exercising is a crucial factor in the ability to learn to self-monitor and regulate exercise intensity. Knowing the safe limits to which patients can exert themselves means they have graduated from the need to be clinically supervised to being independent exercisers.

In the early stages of rehabilitation the exercise leader typically takes a parental role and has more control of the patient, dictating the appropriate exercise intensity. This is done using a combination of HR monitoring, setting specific exercise machine speeds and work rates, observing the patient and using METs to guide the patient. During this period the patient should be made aware of the physical sensations they feel in relation to these set

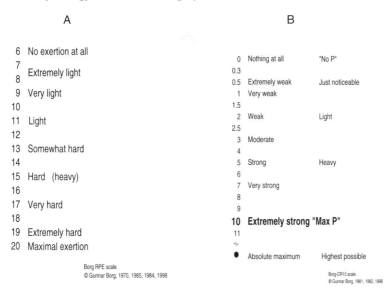

Figure 3.4. (A) Borg's rating of perceived exertion (RPE) and (B) category ratio (CR-10) scales (Borg, 1998).

intensities, which can be rated on a scale of perceived exertion. The most widely and almost exclusively used scales are Borg's (1998) perceived exertion scales (Figure 3.4 A and B). These scales are found in practically every exercise science, sports medicine textbook, practice guidelines and in most scientific publications that involve aerobic exercise or fitness testing procedures. It took over twenty years (from the 1950s to 1970s) for Borg to formulate what was felt to be a 6–20 point rating scale where each point could be related to a relative physiological strain (e.g. %HRmax, %VO$_2$max or blood lactate). It was another 13 years (1970 to 1983) before he validated his category ratio 10-point scale (CR-10; Figure 3.4 B). Borg has continued in recent years to refine the theoretical concept of what he terms psycho-physical scaling (Borg, 1998).

WHICH RPE SCALE SHOULD I USE?

Without going into the detail of the psycho-physics of rating perceived exertion, the RPE (6 to 20) scale was mainly developed around the use of whole body aerobic-type exercise. The CR-10 scale was developed to focus more on rating individual or differentiated perceptions of strain, exertion or pain. Hence, if localised muscle fatigue, pain or breathlessness is the overriding sensation, the CR-10 scale should be used. These more localised and concentrated sensations correspond to an accelerating curvilinear response; e.g. breathlessness grows at a faster rate than does each increment in the stimulus (e.g. exercise workrate). The CR-10 may be the scale of choice with breathless patients. The RPE (6 to 20) is advised in CR because it is moderate submaximal exercise, where muscle and breathing sensations respond in an almost parallel fashion to the exercise stimulus, unlike exercising at higher intensities.

PERCEIVED EXERTION IS MORE THAN USING AN RPE SCALE

Many clinicians will discharge patients based on the rating of perceived exertion (RPE) scale. However, there is another step to be achieved, and that is for patients to be knowledgeable and experienced with the physical sensations, without the rating scale, of the appropriate intensity. The ultimate example of using perceived exertion to control exercise intensity is found in elite endurance athletes who, through their continuous training, have developed a strong sense for pacing. They are able to endure exercise on a very fine line between sustaining their pace and becoming fatigued; physiologists studying bicycle performance have termed this point the 'critical power'. This strong sense, which becomes natural, comes from learning to integrate and judge the sensations arising from the muscles, limb speed and strain, breathing intensity and visual cues of movement (Robertson and Noble, 1997). With regular and frequent exercise, there is no reason why cardiac patients should not be able to develop a strong sense of perceived exertion for controlling safe and effective exercise intensities. The RPE scale should therefore be used as a tool for helping patients become good perceivers of their exertion. The aim of the CR programme is an early but crucial step towards the patient becoming independent in safely and effectively monitoring levels of exertion. This is not just in terms of exercise but in whatever physical activity they perform during daily living, such as gardening, car washing and housework.

VALIDITY AND RELIABILITY OF RATINGS OF PERCEIVED EXERTION

This section focuses on the validity of RPE to represent a given physiological strain. This method may at first seem one which should be regarded with caution. Such cautionary points will first be highlighted, but practical suggestions will be given later to help increase both the validity and reliability when teaching cardiac patients to use RPE. Interestingly, among the first authors to highlight the steps to increasing the validity of patients using RPE were Maresh and Noble (1984). They specifically focus on exercise testing and prescription in cardiac rehabilitation. Noble and Robertson (1996) refer to

Maresh and Noble's (1984) six-point process to increase validity of RPE verbatim. It will be summarised in brief as part of the practical suggestions in teaching the use of RPE, but the reader is recommended to read this landmark text.

As stated in the introduction to this section, the validity of Borg's RPE scales is based on the rationale that a given number and/or verbal descriptor on the scale represents a given relative physiological strain ($\%VO_2max$, $\%HRRmax$, $\%HRmax$ or the lactate or anaerobic threshold) (Noble and Robertson, 1996; Borg, 1998). As illustrated in Figure 3.1 (page 51) and Table 3.1 (page 54), within the main aerobic component of an exercise session, the target RPE for cardiac patients should be 12 to 15 (somewhat hard) on the RPE scale or 3 to 4 (between moderate and strong) on the CR-10 scale. Figure 3.7 (page 78) provides data that closely correspond to these matching targets for HR, oxygen uptake, blood lactate and RPE.

Whaley, *et al.* (1997), however, suggest that in cardiac patients, the target RPE recommendations should be viewed with caution when compared to non-cardiac individuals; they reported a wider range of RPE scores in the cardiac patients at 60% and 80% of HRRmax. Their conclusions suggest that when exercising cardiac patients at a given point on the RPE scale, there would be less certainty that this was the desired physiological level. What this study did not report was whether the validity and reliability of RPE would improve with practice.

It has been demonstrated that an individual's ability to repeat the same intensity for a given RPE improves with practice in both healthy and clinical populations (Eston and Williams, 1988; Buckley, et al., 2000; Buckley, 2003; Buckley, et al., 2004). In many of these studies the variability of the relative inter-individual physiological strain also reduced over repeated trials. In addition to the influence of familiarity on the accuracy of RPE, other factors need to be acknowledged: the mode (production or estimation) in which RPE is used, the psychological status of the exerciser, the social milieu in which the exercise takes place, the ambient environment, the mode of exercise being performed and the effects of medication. There are other factors (age, circadian rhythms, gender and the nutritional state of blood), but those discussed in this chapter are judged to have most relevance to cardiac populations. Practical suggestions for increasing the reliability and validity of RPE will be described once all these key factors that influence RPE have been discussed.

RPE modes

The three modes of using RPE are: *estimation, production* and *preferred* exertion modes. Until 1980, studies evaluating the effectiveness of perceived exertion solely focused on RPE as a dependent response variable, described as estimation mode.

The first published report of RPE being used to actively control intensity, as the independent variable, known as production mode, was that of Smutok, *et al.* (1980). In this study they first assessed participants with a standardised graded exercise treadmill test, where speed was the independent variable and HR and RPE were dependent variables. In two subsequent tests they then asked participants to control treadmill speed from a target RPE that was previously related to a given percentage of maximal HR. A comparison was thus made between HR and treadmill speeds for a given RPE in estimation mode and production mode. RPE was found to reliably elicit the same HR and treadmill speed under production mode compared to the initial estimation mode, but only when the intensity was greater than 80% of maximal HR. This study therefore questioned the validity of RPE to regulate exercise intensity at lower intensities, which are those typically used in clinical populations such as cardiac patients.

Subsequently, Noble (1982) raised concern that the relationship between physiological strain and perceived exertion was altered depending on the mode in which RPE was used. Byrne and Eston (1998) and Whaley, *et al.* (1997) also reported mismatches in the heart rate-RPE relationship in estimation versus production mode protocols in their study involving cardiac patients. This provides a starting point for considering how RPE is taught to patients in order to improve the validity of RPE to represent a given safe and effective physiological strain.

Estimation mode, as stated above, is where RPE is a dependent variable to a given workload. For example, during testing, where the intensity or work rate (e.g. treadmill speed, cycle load or stepping rate) is predetermined and patients are asked to rate on the RPE scale how hard they feel they are working. Another example during an exercise session is where the exercise practitioner specifically dictates the intensity at which the patients exercise and then asks the patients to rate their level of exertion. To assess whether you are asking the patient to use RPE in estimation mode, the following example statement is helpful: '*I am now going to* increase the pace or speed at which you are exercising and then I would like you to rate on the scale how hard an effort you are making.'

Production mode is where RPE is the independent variable. In this case the patient is asked to take command of regulating the exercise intensity (workload) to elicit a predetermined RPE. This can be more difficult during a circuit or exercise to music-type session. This is a scenario where, when there are no machine dials or monitors, it can become more difficult for the exercise leader to exact control over the individual patient's exercise intensity. Other chapters in this text cover the art of good instruction and teaching to ensure the patient is working to the correct intensity. To know if you are asking the patient to use RPE in production mode, the following example statement is helpful: '*I would now like you to* increase the pace or speed at which you are working, so that you work to an RPE of 12 (an effort of between light and somewhat hard).'

In comparing the instructions above for estimation and production mode, respectively, notice the words used in bold above, '*I am now going to* . . . and *I would like you to* . . .'. Furthermore, production mode RPE is when you give instructions to work to a specified RPE. These subtle differences in instructions can make an important distinction about who has the responsibility for controlling the exercise intensity; is it you the practitioner, or is it the patient?

The use of RPE in estimation or production mode should be dependent on where the patient is within the rehabilitation process. Are your patients psychologically and physiologically skilled with their exercise and perceptions of effort to use production mode? These are factors the practitioner needs to assess at each exercise session.

Preferred exertion is where the patients work to an RPE level they prefer. For unconfident or inexperienced anxious patients, this could be at a low rating because of the fear associated with causing an exertion-related cardiac event. In the early stages of rehabilitation this provides patients with some input and gives them some control over their exercise intensity. It has been demonstrated that individuals who have not been active feel more positive about their exercise when working at a moderate compared to a higher intensity (Parfitt and Eston, 1995; Parfitt, *et al.*, 2000). Once it is recognised that the patient has gained confidence, the exercise leader can encourage them to work to higher levels of effort. This fits with the physiological progressions discussed earlier in the section on monitoring HR. When patients are happy working at the appropriate RPE in estimation mode, they can be moved towards using RPE in production mode. The use of RPE in this way ties in well with the important aspect of helping patients attain a sense of mastery, which is beneficial to their mental well-being (Soenstroem, 1984; Stephens, 1988; Buckley, 2003).

RPE, psychological status and social milieu

Psychosocial factors can influence up to 30% of the variability in an RPE score (Dishman and Landy, 1988; Williams and Eston, 1989). Such influences may help to explain the wider variability of RPE, for a given %HRRmax, reported by Whaley, *et al.* (1997) in cardiac compared to non-cardiac individuals. The patients' psychological status has two aspects, which can influence RPE: their state of mental well being and the state of motivation to exercise. The social milieu in which the exercise takes place plays a key role in influencing patients' well-being and motivation to exercise (Dishman, 1994). It is known that following a cardiac event, there can be a concomitant psychological morbidity (Todd, *et al.*, 1992). Individuals with heightened anxiety and depression tend to inflate estimation mode RPE scores compared to those without psychological morbidity (Rejeski, 1981). Furthermore, Kohl and Shea (1988) suggested, though the evidence is equivocal, that individuals with an external locus of control compared to those with an internal locus of control give higher RPEs for a given work rate.

It has been reported that RPE inflation also occurs in individuals with limited experience of exercise fatigue and/or in those inhibited by a social situation (Morgan, 1973; Rejeski, 1981; Morgan, 1994). The inhibiting social situation can include an exercise test, individuals feeling inferior to other patients' abilities in ability, consciousness of body image or physical inferiority, and competitiveness during the exercise session. The effect of psychological status and the presence of disease in modulating RPE scores are not new areas of investigation (Borg and Linderholm, 1970; Morgan, 1973; Morgan, 1994). Borg and Linderholm (1970) found that cardiac patients gave higher RPE values for a given HR compared to age-matched control participants. This greater RPE in the patient group was correlated with the severity of disease. Therefore, not only is RPE used as an aid to monitor exercise intensity, but the RPE values that individuals give may provide cues to the practitioner to consider the patient's psychological state.

Considering all of these issues, changes in RPE over a course of rehabilitation may partially be a function of changes in psychological well being. Nevertheless, for patients to perceive their exercise as getting easier over time, independent of the amount of physiological change, provides positive feedback and motivation towards continued participation through a sense of achievement (Dishman, 1994). Continued participation will secure the longer-term physiological benefits that patients can derive from regular exercise.

RPE and the ambient environment

The ambient environment includes the temperature and humidity of the exercise environment, the effects of water during swimming pool exercise and any audio-visual stimulants. The strongest association of temperature and humidity to RPE is found with skin temperature (Pivarnik and Senay, 1986). When skin temperature is raised, either as result of increased room temperature, humidity or core temperature not being dissipated due to higher humidity, RPE increases for a given work rate.

Music has been demonstrated to dampen perceptions of exertion more than visual distractions like video displays or televisions (Karagheorghis and Terry, 1997; Nethery, 2002). This is important for cardiac patients, where background music could potentially influence patients to over-exert themselves.

Water-based activity has also been shown to be a damper of perceived exertion in light of the following evidence. Movement in water is used therapeutically because it greatly reduces both the gravitational and traction load on skeletal joints, while at the same time providing external resistance (Prins and Cutner, 1999). It is believed to have a soothing interface with the skin and dampens the potential for jerky limb movements (Sukenik, *et al.*, 1999). The presence of water dampens the degree of sensation arising from the muscle spindle and tendon stretch/speed receptors. Water is also a medium for preventing rises in skin temperature. Submersion in water abolishes the

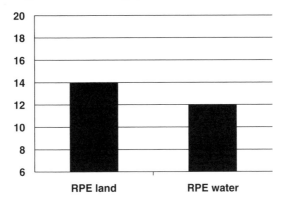

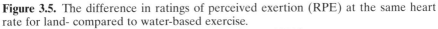

Figure 3.5. The difference in ratings of perceived exertion (RPE) at the same heart rate for land- compared to water-based exercise.
(Adapted from Ueda and Kurokawa, 1995; Green, 1999.)

hydrostatic effect of gravity on circulation, resulting in increased venous return to the heart (Neilsen, *et al.*, 1984). In this environment myocardial work is increased to deal with a greater volume-rate of blood returned to the heart (Meyer and Bucking, 2004). For the coronary heart diseased patient, such hydrostatic changes, together with the dampening of exertion sensations, will increase the likelihood of overexertion and increased myocardial work. Figure 3.5 illustrates a lower RPE for a given heart rate during water-based compared to land-based activity. RPE does not, therefore, represent the same physiological strain in water compared to land (Ueda and Kurokawa, 1995; Green, *et al.*, 1999). This does not mean RPE is invalid during water-based activity: it means, rather, that the target RPE needs to be about two points lower in water- compared to land-based exercise. There is, however, a paucity of research into the cardiorespiratory responses for cardiac patients performing water-based activity.

Mode of exercise

A number of studies have reported variations in the physiological strain at the same RPE when performing different exercises (Eston and Williams, 1988; Thomas, *et al.*, 1995; Zeni, *et al.*, 1996; Buckley, *et al.*, 2000; Moyna, *et al.*, 2001). Table 3.5 summarises these.

The three main explanations for physiological strain differences for a given RPE were that:

- Different modes of exercise each have a mode-specific VO_2max.
- Individuals are likely to be more trained in one activity than another.

Table 3.5. Differences in physiological strain at the same RPE in a variety of exercise machines

Exercise Mode	%HRmax at RPE 13
Treadmill	85%
Stepping machine	75%
Rowing ergometry	75%
Cross-country ski machine	73%
Cycle ergometer	69%

(Adapted from: Thomas, *et al.*, 1995; Zeni, *et al.*, 1996; Eston and Williams, 1988; Moyna, *et al.*, 2001; Buckley, *et al.*, 2000.)

- The motor-skill familiarisation and types of muscle movements recruited to perform specific activities lead to different energy usage economies.

These three factors demonstrate the sensitivity of RPE in detecting exercise mode differences, summarised in Table 3.5, which relate to the concepts of specificity of training and training status. The concept of specificity of training is that training adaptations occur only in those muscles or individual muscle units involved in the activity (Astrand, *et al.*, 2003). Typically, the average person more frequently uses muscle units for walking and stepping actions compared to cycling, rowing and cross-country skiing. In healthy and cardiac populations, a specific muscle unit that is more frequently used (trained) results in a lowered production of lactate for a given VO_2 or heart rate compared with a less trained muscle unit (Ekblom, *et al.*, 1968; Sullivan, *et al.*, 1989; Meyer, *et al.*, 1990; Goodman, *et al.*, 1999).

Figure 3.6 illustrates how RPE is independent of training status as it does not change for a given blood lactate. Both %HRmax or %VO_2max at a given RPE alter with a change in training status. RPE may therefore be more closely linked to blood lactate than %HRmax and %VO_2max, which is a function of muscle metabolism. In practical terms this means that for progressing exercise intensity, by working to the same RPE, the patient's exercise intensity will be automatically adjusted for both the expected increase in VO_2max and work rate that corresponds to the lactate threshold. This was not true for HR, as explained earlier in this chapter, where over time it should be progressed towards the upper end of the recommended target zone. Figure 3.7 (p. 78) summarises the link between the typical target RPE of 13 (somewhat hard) and HR, VO_2 and blood lactate.

Beta-blocking medication

Beta-blockers, unless contraindicated, are now standardised prescription in the UK and the USA following myocardial infarction (Brand, *et al.*, 1995;

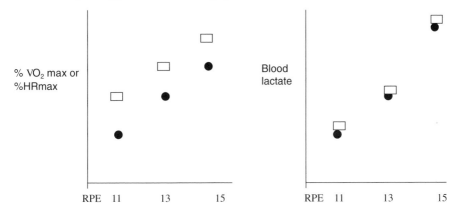

Figure 3.6. RPE, %VO$_2$ max, %HRmax and blood lactate in trained (open boxes) and untrained (black circles) individuals.
(Adapted from the summary of findings of: Berry, *et al.*, 1989; Boutcher, *et al.*, 1989; Briswalter and Delignieres, 1997; Ekblom and Goldbarg, 1971; Held, *et al.*, 1997; Held and Marti, 1999; Hetzler, *et al.*, 1991; Hill, *et al.*, 1987; Kang, *et al.*, 1996; Seip, *et al.*, 1991; Swaine, *et al.*, 1995; Travlos and Marisi, 1996.)

Department of Health: National Service Framework for Coronary Heart Disease, 2000). These guidelines recommend that patients be prescribed beta-blockers for at least 12 months following myocardial infarction. This means that most post-MI patients attending cardiac rehabilitation will require an exercise prescription that respects the effects of beta-blockade, including: an altered cardio-respiratory response, changes in physical performance capability, slowed oxygen kinetics and potential side effects such as postural hypotension (Hughson and Smyth, 1983; Reents, 2000).

The year 1979 appears to be a watershed for research published on the potential interactions between beta-blockade and perceived exertion. Three studies (Davies and Sargeant, 1979; Sjoberg, *et al.*, 1979; van Herwarden, 1979) reported that the use of beta-blockade did not affect perceived exertion. One study did report an increase in RPE with the administration of beta-blockade (Pearson, *et al.*, 1979). However, this study involved healthy participants, where the other studies involved either hypertensive or myocardial infarction patients. The validity of studying the effects of beta-blockade on normotensive and non-cardiac diseased patients is thus questioned.

Wilcox, *et al.* (1984) reported that in the acute stages of first administering beta-blockers, RPE was modulated upward for a given exercise intensity. It is therefore important to consider the wash-in period of these medications during research and during the practice of exercise prescription when patients are either first given medication or have medication changed. The review by Eston and Connolly (1996) was very clear to point out that studies on RPE

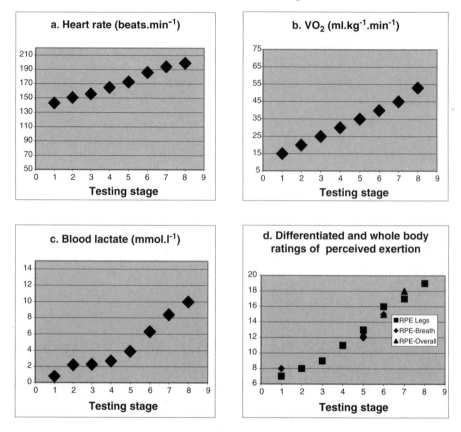

Figure 3.7. Heart rate (a), oxygen uptake (b), blood lactate, (c) RPE and (d) responses to an incremental maximal cycle ergometer test.

These data correspond with the studies referenced in Figure 3.6. Take note of the RPE values of 12 to 13, at testing stages 4 to 5, corresponding to the point where blood lactate has risen in an accelerating fashion (the lactate threshold). For this individual this point was at 80% of HRmax and 64% VO₂max.

(Buckley JP and Whyte G (Oct. 2003) Unpublished data: British Olympic Medical Institute, London.)

and beta-blockade involved three different types of participants: healthy individuals, patients with hypertension and patients with angina or a previous myocardial infarction. A further consideration is that a variety of makes and types of beta-blockade (e.g. *atenolol, bisoprolol, celiprolol, metoprolol, practolol, propranolol*) were used in the four studies noted above.

The majority of studies have shown that beta-blockade does not interact with RPE, but with two key exceptions: (1). When the exercise lasts for more than 60 minutes and (2). When exercise is performed at higher relative intensities (>~65% VO_2 max) (Eston and Connolly, 1996; Noble and Robertson, 1996; Head, *et al.*, 1997; Borg, 1998; Liu, *et al.*, 2000). The latter exception appears to have been a function of the type of beta-blocker prescribed, and with some brands RPE is unchanged for a given %VO_2 max, regardless of intensity. These levels of intensity (>65% max) and duration (>60 minutes) represent more advanced limits of exercise prescription for cardiovascular patients (ACSM, 1994, 2000; BACR, 1995; AACVPR, 2004). The majority of patients in phase III and IV rehabilitation programmes will exercise at the low to moderate level of exercise. Other interactions between RPE and beta-blockade have also been dependent on whether the ratings were measured as overall, central (cardio-pulmonary) or peripheral/local (muscle) sensations (see Figure 3.7) and whether or not the beta-blocker was a cardioselective drug. It has been shown that non-selective compared to cardioselective beta-blocking medications have more influence in reducing blood flow to pulmonary tissues and skeletal muscle (British National Formulary, 2004), but that all types dampen fat metabolism (Eston and Connolly, 1996; Head, *et al.*, 1997; Lamont, *et al.*, 1997). Thus, there could be an increased perception of pulmonary effort due to an increased demand on carbohydrate and decreased supply of oxygen and free fatty acids to the skeletal muscle. Muscle fatigue during prolonged low-to-moderate intensity exercise is linked to reductions in carbohydrate reserves (Newsolme, *et al.*, 1992). Cardioselective beta-blockers (e.g. atenolol) have less effect on blocking beta-receptors in pulmonary tissue and skeletal muscle. It can therefore be seen why both the effect of reduced fatty acid metabolism and non-cardioselective beta-blockade may cause an increased local/peripheral perception of effort. Furthermore, during prolonged (>60 minutes) and/or higher intensity (>65% VO_2 max) exercise there will be an increased susceptibility to an earlier onset of muscle fatigue due to increased reliance on limited carbohydrate substrates.

Duration of exercise has been regarded as a modulator of RPE whether under beta-blockade or not, from the effects of reductions in carbohydrate energy substrates, increased body temperature and the psychological concept of duration-fatigue (Potteiger and Weber, 1994; Kang, *et al.*, 1996; Head, *et al.*, 1997; Utter, *et al.*, 1997, 1999; Borg, 1998).

SUMMARY OF KEY POINTS FOR THE EFFECTIVE USE OF RPE

The following points include the key instruction statements recommended by Maresh and Noble (1984).

1. Make sure the patient understands what an RPE is. Before using the scale see if they can grasp the concept of sensing the exercise responses (breathing, muscle movement/strain, joint movement/speed).

2. Anchor the perceptual range, which includes relating to the fact that no exertion at all is sitting still, and maximal exertion is a theoretical concept of pushing the body to its absolute physical limits. Patients should then be exposed to differing levels of exercise intensity (as in an incremental test or during an exercise session) so as to understand what the various levels on the scale feel like. Just giving them one or two points on the scale to aim for will probably result in a great deal of variability.

3. Use the above points to explain the nature of the scale and explain that the patient should consider both the verbal descriptor and the numerical value. Many practitioners simply state, 'choose a number'. That is the last thing they should do. They should first concentrate on the sensations arising from the activity, look at the scale to see which verbal descriptor relates to the effort they are experiencing and then link it to the numerical value.

4. Make sure the patient is not just concentrating on singular sensations, known as differentiated ratings (see Figure 3.7). For aerobic exercise they should pool all sensations to give one rating. If there is an overriding sensation, note the differentiated rating for this. Differentiated ratings can be used during muscular strength activity or where exercise is limited more by breathlessness or leg pain, and not cardiac limitations, as in the case pulmonary or peripheral vascular disease, respectively.

5. Confirm that there is no right or wrong answer: it is what the patient perceives. There are three important cases where the patient may give an incorrect rating:

   a. When the patient already has a preconceived idea about what exertion level is elicited by a specific activity (Borg, 1998). He/she is not aware that what is required is to rate the amount of effort at this very moment, not what they think a typical level of exertion is for that activity.

   b. When patients are asked to recall the exercise and give a rating. Similar to heart rate, RPEs should be taken while the patient is actually engaged in the movements, not after they have finished or in the break between stations.

   c. Simply pleasing the exercise practitioner by stating what should be the appropriate level is a regular observation in the author's experience. This is typically the case when patients are told ahead of time (e.g. in education sessions or during the warm-up) to what RPE level they should work. In the early stages of rehabilitation, the patient's exercise intensity should be set by HR or workrate (e.g. in METs), and patients need to learn to match their RPE reliably to this level in estimation mode. Once it has been established that the patient's rating concurs with the target heart rate or MET level reliably, moving them on to production mode can be considered.

6. Keep RPE scales in full view at all times (e.g. on each machine or circuit station) and keep reminding patients throughout their exercise session to think about what sort of sensations they have while making their

judgement rating. It is known that endurance athletes in a race situation work very hard mentally to concentrate (cognitively associate) on their sensations in order to regulate their pace effectively (Morgan, 2000).

ESTIMATED METABOLIC EQUIVALENTS

The metabolic equivalent (MET) is widely used in cardiovascular population exercise guidelines as a means of quantifying the energy demands of physical activity. It relates the rate of the body's oxygen uptake (VO_2) for a given activity as a multiple of an individual's resting VO_2. At rest an individual's basal VO_2 is on average 3.5 millilitres of oxygen per minute for every kilogram of body mass ($ml.kg^{-1}.min^{-1}$).

One MET has therefore been set to equal a VO_2 of $3.5 ml.kg^{-1}.min^{-1}$. By measuring the VO_2 of an activity an MET value can then be assigned to it. For example, if a person walks at ~5 kph ($3.0 mph = 11.6 ml.kg^{-1}.min^{-1}$) on the flat, the oxygen cost will be:

$11.6 ml.kg^{-1}.min^{-1}$
If 1 MET equals a VO_2 of $3.5 ml.kg^{-1}.min^{-1}$
then a VO_2 of $11.6 ml.kg^{-1}.min^{-1}$ = 3.3 METs

The full calculation for this can be found in the ACSM (2000) guidelines for exercise testing and prescription.

Variability in estimated METs

Ainsworth, *et al.* (1993) have compiled an extensive compendium on the estimated MET values for a variety of physical activities. It is important to recognise that these values are estimates, which means that each individual patient could be working above or below this estimate. The variability of the estimate depends on the simplicity or complexity of the movements. For example, the variability of pedalling an exercise cycle ergometer will likely be less than that of stepping or walking. The motor skill involved in cycle ergometry is fixed by the motion of the pedal crank and mainly involves the legs. Stepping and walking require the individual to balance and use arm and trunk motions, which can vary much more than cycling.

In cardiac rehabilitation, the MET values from the patients' exercise ECG stress test are typically reported. These data provide the exercise leader with information of both intensity and functional capacity. It should be noted, if the ETT is carried out using a motorised treadmill, how much the MET value can be altered by the patient holding on to the handrail. Astrand (1982) reported that when walking on the treadmill with hands on the rail, the VO_2 was as much as $9 ml.kg^{-1}.min^{-1}$ (2.6 METs) lower than walking with hands free. Most patients attending an exercise ECG stress test will hold on to the rail because they are typically unfamiliar with treadmill exercise and are not used to a moving platform. In addition treadmill walking mechanics are very different from floor walking, making direct comparison of floor to treadmill walking questionable.

Using the ACSM (2000) equations or data from Ainsworth, *et al.* (1993), MET values can also be estimated from submaximal protocols recommended for assessing functional capacity in cardiac patients in the UK, including: step tests, shuttle walks and cycle ergometry (BACR, 1995; Tobin and Thow, 1999; ACPICR, 2003; Fowler, *et al.*, 2005).

For box-stepping exercise performed in healthy young individuals, the variability (based on the 95% limits of agreement) in the estimated versus actual MET (VO_2) values was found to be up to 1.3 METs (4.5 ml.kg^{-1}.min^{-1}) (Buckley, *et al.*, 2004). This work on box stepping is presently being replicated by Buckley with older individuals and cardiovascular patients as participants. It is anticipated that such variability would not be less than that found in the younger, healthier and more active individuals reported above. Another step test being suggested for rehabilitation settings is the Chester step test (CST) (Sykes, 1995). The CST is a sub-max, multi-stage test lasting for 10 minutes with a choice of four step heights. It has been shown to be valid in the estimation of aerobic capacity in a non-clinical sample with a range of fitness levels (Sykes and Roberts, 2004). This novel test would appear to be promising in the CR setting. The estimated MET values for step heights and stepping rates that would be appropriate to cardiac populations are summarised in Table 3.6.

The assessment recommended by Tobin and Thow (1999) and SIGN (2002), which is adapted from Singh, *et al.* (1992), provides walking speeds for each

Table 3.6. Estimated metabolic equivalents (METs) for box stepping on a 6-inch, 8-inch and 10-inch step

*Stepping rate (steps·min^{-1})	**Metronome setting (beats·min^{-1})	METs for a 6-inch step	METs for an 8-inch step	METs for a 10-inch step
14	56	2.8	3.4	3.9
16	64	3.2	3.8	4.4
18	72	3.6	4.3	5.0
20	80	4	4.8	5.5
22	88	4.4	5.3	6.1
24	96	4.8	5.8	6.6
26	104	5.2	6.2	7.2
28	112	5.6	6.7	7.7
30	120	6	7.2	8.3

*One step, commencing from both feet on the ground, constitutes each foot stepping up and then each foot stepping down. Each foot movement is paced with each beat of the **Metronome; four beats of the metronome equal a one-step cycle.
(Adapted from the ACSM, 2000, p. 305.)

testing stage, which can be converted into METs. An important point to remember is that the testing stages are only one minute in duration, which means that it is more difficult to determine the MET level that an individual can actually sustain. Furthermore, in each of these one-minute periods, the heart rate and RPE responses will not have had time to plateau, to associate the MET level with the corresponding HR or RPE. Box 3.1 provides the shuttle walk test protocol (SIGN, 2002).

Box 3.1 Shuttle walk test protocol

Equipment required

- Calibrated cassette player and shuttle walk test tape.
- Two marker cones and non-slippery, flat walking surface at least 10 metres in length.
- Heart rate monitor with record facilities and adjustable upper alarm limits.

Protocol

- Each subject should be screened by a member of the cardiac rehabilitation team for any exclusion criteria before proceeding.
- Place two cones exactly 9 metres apart, thus allowing the subjects to walk 10 metres when they go round the cone at each end of each shuttle.
- Subjects then listen to the instructions on the audio cassette. These should be repeated verbally to ensure they understand what is expected during the test.
- Subjects walk around the 10-metre course aiming to be turning at the first marker cone when the first audio signal is given, and turning at the second cone at the end of the next audio signal.
- Subjects should be accompanied around the first level of the test to help them keep pace with the audio signals. Thereafter the operator stands mid-way between the two marker cones offering advice on completion of a level: '*Walk a bit faster now if you can.*'
- Progression to the next level of difficulty is indicated by a triple bleep which lets the subject know that an increase in walking speed is required.
- The full test comprises 12 levels each of one minute duration with walking speeds that rise incrementally from 1.2 miles per hour (1.9 km per hour) to 5.3 miles per hour (8.5 km per hour).
- The test is completed at 12 minutes or if one of the termination criteria are met.

Termination criteria

- any anginal symptoms or feeling too breathless to continue;
- feeling dizzy or faint;
- leg pain limiting further exercise;
- achieved level of perceived exertion ≤15 Borg scale;
- achieved heart rate ≥85% predicted (detected by audible upper alarm limit);
- failure to meet the speed requirement of the test – subject more than half a metre from the cone when the bleep sounds.

Following the test

- Subjects should continue to walk slowly round the course a further four times to avoid any syncopal attacks associated with abrupt cessation of exercise.
- Subjects are then seated and asked to confirm their limiting symptom.
- Record total distance walked, heart rate and perceived exertion for each level completed, peak heart rate and reason for termination.
- If subjects have fully recovered after 10 minutes then no further action is required. If they report continuing breathlessness or angina then a further rest period should follow during which they may receive sub-lingual nitrates, have an ECG or be seen by a doctor as appropriate.

Singh, *et al.*, 1992. Reproduced with permission (SIGN, 2002).

Table 3.7. Estimated metabolic equivalents (METs) for each stage of a shuttle-walking assessment

Test stage	Walking speed (km/hr)	VO_2 (ml·kg^{-1}·min^{-1})	METS
1	1.8	6.5	1.9
2	2.41	7.5	2.1
3	3.03	8.6	2.4
4	3.63	9.6	2.7
5	4.25	10.6	3.0
6	4.86	11.6	3.3
7	5.47	12.6	3.6
8	6.08	13.7	3.9
9	6.69	14.7	4.2
*10	7.31	27.9	8.0
11	7.92	30.0	8.6
12	8.53	32.0	9.1

*Note the large increase in METs as the speed between 6.5 to 7.5 kph is the threshold between walking and running.
(Adapted from Singh, *et al.* (1992) and Tobin and Thow (1999) applying equations from ACSM, 2000 p. 303.)

Table 3.8. Cycle ergometer estimated metabolic equivalents (METs)

Body Weight (kg)	Body Weight (lbs)	25 Watts	50 Watts	75 Watts	100 Watts	125 Watts	150 Watts	175 Watts	200 Watts
50	110	3.0	5.1	6.6	8.2	9.7	11.3	12.8	14.3
60	132	2.3	4.6	5.9	7.1	8.4	9.7	11.0	12.3
70	154	2.1	4.2	5.3	6.4	7.5	8.6	9.7	10.8
80	176	2.0	3.9	4.9	5.9	6.8	7.8	8.8	9.7
90	198	2.0*	3.7	4.6	5.4	6.3	7.1	8.0	8.9
100	220	2.0*	3.5	4.3	5.1	5.9	6.6	7.4	8.2

*It is felt difficult to estimate the MET value when an activity is less than 2 METs.
(Adapted from the ACSM, 2000 p. 304.)

The best way to set an initial intensity from this protocol is to take the peak MET value attained during the test and then determine what MET value represents 50–60% of this peak (Peak METs × 0.5 or Peak METs × 0.6). Then guide the patient's activities that equate to this MET value as outlined by Ainsworth, *et al.* (1993), ACSM (2000), AACVPR (2004) or BACR (1995, 2001). Table 3.7 summarises the MET values for the walking speeds in this protocol recommended by Tobin and Thow (1999) and SIGN (2002).

Similar principles for cycle ergometry can be applied as with the stepping and walking above. Cycle ergometers with accurate readings in Watts are required with MET values summarised in Table 3.8.

Rowing ergometry, especially the Concept II models, is now being used in rehabilitation settings (Buckley, *et al.*, 1999a). The oxygen uptake of rowing on the Concept II ergometer can be determined using the regression equations developed by Lakomy and Lakomy (1993). Table 3.9 summarises the MET values for the Concept II rowing ergometer speeds, which can be determined from the machine's monitor read-out expressed as the 500-metre split time.

OBSERVATION

Observation of the exerciser by the exercise leader and assistants is a vital aspect of monitoring. The leader and assistants should monitor the CR exerciser continuously for quality of movement, excessive sweating, shortness of breath, skin colour and general fatigue. As part of the teaching skills the leader and assistants should scan the group and also maintain face and eye contact. These can be indicators of overexertion and a need to adapt or reduce exercise intensity. It is important that there is continuity of exercise leader to ensure that the leader/s becomes familiar with the participants and how they react to exercise. (Chapter 7 will explore observation further.)

Table 3.9. Estimated metabolic equivalents (METs) for a given rowing on a Concept-II Ergometer. Rowing speed is described as the 500-meter split time, which is the largest value displayed on the ergometer console

Rowing speed 500-m split time	60 kg 132 lbs	70 kg 154 lbs	80 kg 176 lbs	90 kg 198 lbs	100 kg 220 lbs
4:30	2.10	2.0	2.0	2.0	2.0
4:15	2.57	2.2	2.0	2.0	2.0
4:00	3.38	2.9	2.54	2.25	2.03
3:40	4.29	3.67	3.21	2.86	2.57
3:25	4.76	4.08	3.57	3.17	2.86
3:15	5.24	4.49	3.93	3.49	3.14
3:05	5.48	4.69	4.11	3.65	3.29
3:00	6.19	5.31	4.64	4.13	3.71
2:55	7.14	6.12	5.36	4.76	4.29
2:45	7.81	6.69	5.86	5.21	4.69
2:38	8.57	7.35	6.43	5.71	5.14
2:30	8.86	7.59	6.64	5.90	5.31
2:28	9.52	8.16	7.14	6.35	5.71
2:25	10.00	8.57	7.50	6.67	6.00
2:21	10.86	9.31	8.14	7.24	6.61
2:18	11.52	9.88	8.64	7.68	6.91
2:15	12.24	10.49	9.18	8.16	7.34
2:12	12.86	11.02	9.64	8.57	7.71
2:10	13.33	11.43	10.00	8.89	8.00
2:07	14.95	12.82	11.21	9.97	8.97
2:00	17.00	14.57	12.74	11.33	10.20

(Adapted from Lakomy and Lakomy, 1993.)

INTEGRATING THE USE OF HEART RATE, RPE, METS AND OBSERVATION

As discussed in the preceding sections, at times there are limitations to the reliability and validity of using either HR, RPE, observation and METs alone to control or monitor exercise intensity in the cardiac patient. Furthermore, the patient's psychological state may be an important factor that holds back or advances too quickly the patient from exercising at the physiologically beneficial intensity. Figure 3.8 summarises these four important facets to guiding the patient towards the appropriate intensity, eventually with them taking command. The RPE provides a channel through which the patient's psychological status influences the appropriate exercise intensity.

In the initial stages of rehabilitation, if an MET value and HR are known from an ETT, to show the intensity at which any critical cardiac events occur, these should be used to guide exercise intensity. RPE should be used immediately to link with these, but its reliability to represent these levels should be

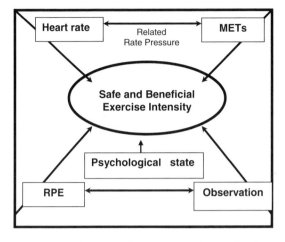

Figure 3.8. Framework of the integrated components in monitoring exercise intensity in cardiac patient rehabilitation.

assessed. It has been reported that patients tend to inflate their RPE in an initial exercise ETT compared to subsequent exercise at the same intensity in the CR exercise class, with only a few days separating the two sessions (Buckley, *et al.*, 2000). If the exercise sessions involve the use of exercise machines, then either HR or METs, relative to the peak measurements from the exercise test, can be used to set intensity. If the exercise is a class, circuit or home-based activity then HR will be the obvious choice initially, but giving patients advice about what activities they can or should do based on the MET value is an important adjunct. Models of good practice for home-based programmes involve either having a few instructional sessions with the patients as part of an outpatient clinic before patients exercise at home, and/or supporting this with a video (see the British Heart Foundation: www.bhf.org.uk) or an individualised home programme using Physiotools (2005), etc.

For monitoring exercise subsequent to more practical assessments (step test, cycle test, shuttle walk) the appropriate level should be one that equates to the intensity that the patient can sustain. These tests are designed to raise intensity incrementally to a level which elicits an HR of ≤60%HRRmax or 75%HRmax and an RPE of 13 to 15 as per the upper limit guidelines in Table 3.1 (see page 54). From the MET level or 75%HRmax that corresponds with the end of the test, subsequent exercise intensities can be monitored relative to this. This principle can be used even when patients are beta-blocked, but the HR has to be adjusted, as recommended in Table 3.3 (see pages 61–2).

The cue to progressing intensity in all the above cases is when, for a given work rate, there is a noticeable decrease in both HR (>5 beats.min^{-1}) and RPE (≥1.5 RPE points). If there is a noticeable decrease in HR there should be a nding decrease in RPE. If there is not a corresponding decrease in ⌐ with HR, this is a sign that the accurate use and understanding of RPE is yet to be established. In addition, the skills of the exercise leader to observe the participant are vital in delivering safe and effective CR.

Finally, it is important that patients learn to self-monitor changes by reporting and/or associating their improved levels of fitness relative to changes they experience in activities of daily living (away from the structured class). When patients are able to recognise their changes and benefits, they are better able to judge their own level of functional health or change of symptoms that could occur in the future.

SUMMARY

CR exercise and monitoring require a sound knowledge of the complex interaction of many physiological and psychological factors. In addition, observation by the exercise leader is a vital element in monitoring an exercise test or training session. This chapter provides the underpinning knowledge to prescribe and monitor the CR exercise class. In addition, strategies to help teach and explain self-monitoring to patients are addressed.

REFERENCES

Ades, P.A., Waldmann, M.L., Meyer, W.L., Brown, K.A., Poehlman, E.T., Pendlebury, W.W., *et al.* (1996) Skeletal muscle and cardiovascular adaptations to exercise conditioning in older coronary patients. *Circulation*, **94**, 323–30.

Ainsworth, B.E., Haskell, W.L., Leon, A.S., Jacobs, D.R., Jr, Montoye, H.J., Sallis, J.F., *et al.* (1993) Compendium of physical activities: Classification of energy costs of human physical activities. *Medicine and Science in Sports Exercise*, **25**, 71–80.

Ajisaka, R., Watanabe, S., Eda, K., Sakamoto, K., Saitou, T., Yamaguchi, I., *et al.* (2000) Hemodynamic and thermal responses to a 30-minute constant-workload aerobic exercise in middle- or old-aged patients with cardiovascular diseases. *Japanese Circulation Journal*, **64**, 370–6.

American Association of Cardiovascular and Pulmonary Rehabilitation (AACPR) (2004) *Guidelines for Cardiac Rehabilitation Programs*, 4th edn, Human Kinetics, Champaign, IL.

American College of Sports Medicine (ACSM) (1994) Position Stand: Exercise for patients with coronary artery disease. *Medicine and Science in Sports and Exercise*, **26**, I–V.

American College of Sports Medicine (ACSM) (1998) Position stand: The recommended quantity and quality of exercise for developing and maintaining cardiorespiratory and muscular strength and flexibility in healthy adults. *Medicine and Science in Sports and Exercise*, **30**, 975–91.

American College of Sports Medicine (ACSM) (2000) *Guidelines for Exercise Testing and Prescription*, 6th edn, Lippincott, Williams and Wilkins, Baltimore, MD.

Association of Chartered Physiotherapists Interested in Cardiac Rehabilitation (ACPICR) (2003) *Standards for the Exercise Component of Phase III Cardiac Rehabilitation*, The Chartered Society of Physiotherapy, London.

Astrand, P-O. (1982) How to conduct and evaluate an exercise stress test. In *International Approaches to Pulmonary Disease. International exchange of information rehabilitation* (ed. I. Kass), Monograph 18, World Rehabilitation Fund Inc., New York.

Astrand, P-O., Christensen, E.H. (1964) Aerobic work capacity. In *Oxygen in the Animal Organism* (eds F. Dickens, E. Neil and W.F. Widdas), Pergamon Press, New York, pp. 295.

Astrand, P-O., Rhyming, I. (1954) A nomogram for calculation of aerobic capacity from pulse rate during submaximal work. *Journal of Applied Physiology*, **7**, 218.

Astrand, I., Astrand, P-O., Hallback, I., Kilborn, A. (1973) Reduction in maximal oxygen uptake with age. *Journal of Applied Physiology*, **14**, 562–6.

Astrand, P-O., Rodahl, K., Dahl, H.A., Stromme, S.B. (2003) *Textbook of Work Physiology: Physiological bases of exercise*, 4th edn, Human Kinetics, Champaign, IL.

Berry, M.J., Weyrich, A.S., Robergs, R.A., Krause, K.M., Ingallis, C.P. (1989) Ratings of perceived exertion in individuals with varying fitness levels during walking and running. *European Journal of Applied Physiology and Occupational Physiology*, **58**, 494–9.

Bodner, M.E., Rhodes, E.C. (2000) A review of the concept of the heart rate deflection point. *Sports Medicine*, **30**, 31–46.

Borg, G.A.V. (1998) *Borg's Perceived Exertion and Pain Scales*, Human Kinetics, Champaign, IL.

Borg, G., Linderholm, H. (1970) Exercise performance and perceived exertion in patients with coronary insufficiency, arterial hypertension and vasoregulatory asthenia. *Acta Medica Scandinavica*, **187**, 17–26.

Boutcher, S.H., Seip, R.L., Hetzler, R.K., Pierce, E.F., Snead, D., Weltman, A. (1989) The effects of specificity of training on the rating of perceived exertion at the lactate threshold. *European Journal of Applied Physiology*, **59**, 365–9.

Brand, D.A., Newcomer, L.N., Freiburger, A., Tian, H. (1995) Practices compared with practice guidelines: Use of beta-blockade after acute myocardial infarction. *Journal of the American College of Cardiology*, **26**, 1432–6.

Briswalter, J., Delignieres, D. (1997) Influence of exercise duration on perceived exertion during controlled locomotion. *Perceptual and Motor Skills*, **85**, 17–18.

British Association for Cardiac Rehabilitation (BACR) (1995) *Guidelines for Cardiac Rehabilitation*, Blackwell Science, Oxford.

British National Formulary (2004) *British Medical Association and the Royal Pharmaceutical Society.* London: 44.

Buckley, J., Davis, J., Simpson, T. (1999a) Cardio-respiratory responses to rowing ergometry and treadmill exercise soon after myocardial infarction. *Medicine and Science in Sports and Exercise*, **31**, 1721–6.

Buckley, J., Holmes, J., Mapp, G. (1999b) *Exercise on Prescription: Cardiovascular activity for health*, Butterworth Heinemann, Oxford.

Buckley, J.P. (2003) Ratings of perceived exertion in the assessment and prescription of exercise. PhD thesis. University of Staffordshire, Keele.

Buckley, J.P., Eston, R.G., Sim, J. (2000) Ratings of perceived exertion in Braille: Validity and reliability in production mode. *British Journal of Sports Medicine*, **34**, 297–302.

Buckley, J.P., Sim, J., Eston, R.G., Hession, R., Fox, R. (2004) Reliability and validity of measures taken during the Chester step test to predict aerobic power and to prescribe aerobic exercise. *British Journal of Sports Medicine*, **38**, 197–205.

Buckley, P., Whyte, G. (Oct. 2003) Unpublished data: British Olympic Medical Institute, London.

Byrne, C., Eston, R.G. (1998) Use of ratings of perceived exertion to regulate exercise intensity: A study using effort estimation and effort production. *Journal of Sports Sciences*, **16**, 15–16 (abstract).

Cachovan, M., Marees, H., Kunitsch, G. (1976) Influence of interval training on the physical capacity and peripheral circulation in patients with intermittent claudication. *Zeitschrift Kardiologie*, **65**, 54–67.

Carlson, J.J., Norman, G.J., Feltz, D.L., Franklin, B.A., Johnson, J.A., Locke, S.K. (2001) Self-efficacy, psychosocial factors, and exercise behavior in traditional versus modified cardiac rehabilitation. *Journal of Cardiopulmonary Rehabilitation*, **21**, 363–73.

Cheatham, C.C., Mahon, A.D., Brown, J.D., Bolster, D.R. (2000) Cardiovascular responses during prolonged exercise at ventilatory threshold in boys and men. *Medicine and Science in Sports and Exercise*, **32**, 1080–7.

Christensen, E.H. (1931) in (2003) *Physical training. Textbook of work physiology; physiological bases of exercise*, 4th edn (eds P-O. Astrand, K. Rodahl, H.A. Dahl and S.B. Stromme), Human Kinetics Champaign, IL, p. 315.

Conconi, F., Ferrari, M., Ziglio, P.G., Droghetti, P., Codeca, L. (1982) Determination of the anaerobic threshold by a noninvasive field test in runners. *Journal of Applied Physiology*, **52**, 869–73.

Cooper, C.B. (2001) Exercise in chronic pulmonary disease: aerobic exercise prescription. *Medicine and Science in Sports and Exercise*, **33** (7) supplement S643–6 Review.

Coplan, N.L., Gleim, G.W., Nicholas, J.A. (1986) Principles of exercise prescription for patients with coronary artery disease. *American Heart Journal*, **112**(1), 145–9.

Coyle, E.F., Gonzalez-Alonso, J. (2001) Cardiovascular drift during prolonged exercise: New perspectives. *Exercise and Sport Science Reviews*, **29**, 88–92.

Davies, C.T., Sargeant, A.J. (1979) The effects of atropine and practolol on the perception of exertion during treadmill exercise. *Ergonomics*, **22**, 1141–6.

Day, W. (2003) Women and cardiac rehabilitation: A review of the literature. *Contemporary Nurse*, **16**, 92–101.

Department of Health (2000) National Service Framework for Coronary Heart Disease Modern Standards and Service Models [online] available from http://www.doh.gov.uk/nsf/coronary [accessed 11 Nov 2002].

DeVan, A.E., Lacy, B.K., Cortez-Cooper, M.Y., Tanaka, H. (2004) Post-exercise palpation of pulse rates: Its applicability to trained individuals. *Medicine and Science in Sports and Exercise*, **36**(5), supplement S4 (Abstract).

Dishman, R. (1994) *Advances in Exercise Adherence*, Human Kinetics, Champaign, IL.

Dishman, R.K., Landy, F.J. (1998) Psychological factors and prolonged exercise in *Perspectives in Exercise Science and Sports Medicine* (eds D.R. Lamb and R. Murray), Benchmark Press, Indianapolis, IN, pp. 281–355.

Edwards, H.T., Brouha, L., Johnson, R.T. (1939) Effects de l'entrainment sur le taux de l'acide lactique sainguin aucours du travail musculaire. *Travail Human*, **8**, 1–9.

Ehsani, A.A., Martin, W.H., 3rd, Heath, G.W., Coyle, E.F. (1982) Cardiac effects of prolonged and intense exercise training in patients with coronary artery disease. *American Journal of Cardiology*, **50**, 246–54.

Ekblom, B., Goldbarg, A.N. (1971) The influence of physical training and other factors on the subjective rating of perceived exertion. *Acta Physiologica Scandinavica*, **83**, 399–406.

Ekblom, B., Astrand, P.-O., Saltin, B., Stenberg, J., Wallstrom, B. (1968) Effect of training on circulatory response to exercise. *Journal of Applied Physiology*, **24**, 518–28.

Eston, R.G., Connolly, D. (1996) The use of ratings of perceived exertion for exercise prescription in patients receiving β-blocker therapy. *Sports Medicine*, **21**, 176–90.

Eston, R.G., Williams, J.G. (1988) Reliability of ratings of perceived exertion for regulation of exercise intensity. *British Journal of Sports Medicine*, **22**, 153–5.

Fowler, S.J., Singh, S.J., Revill, S. (2005) Reproducibility and validity of the incremental shuttle walking test in patients following coronary artery bypass surgery. *Physiotherapy*, **91**, 22–7.

Froelicher, V.F., Myers, J.N. (2000) *Exercise and the Heart*. WB Saunders, Pittsburgh, PA.

Gobel, F.L., Norstrom, L.A., Nelson, R.R., Jorgensen, C.R., Wang, Y. (1978) The rate-pressure product as an index of myocardial oxygen consumption during exercise in patients with angina pectoris. *Circulation*, **57**, 549–56.

Goodman, J.M., Pallandi, D.V., Reading, J.R., Plyley, M.J., Liu, P.P., Kavanagh, T. (1999) Central and peripheral adaptations after 12 weeks of exercise training in post-coronary artery bypass surgery patients. *Journal of Cardiopulmonary Rehabilitation*, **19**, 144–50.

Green, J.M., Michael, T., Solomon, A.H. (1999) The validity of ratings of perceived exertion for cross-modal regulation of swimming intensity. *Sports Medicine and Physical Fitness*, **39**, 207–12.

Head, A., Maxwell, S., Kendall, M.J. (1997) Exercise metabolism in healthy volunteers taking celiprolol, atenolol, and placebo. *British Journal of Sports Medicine*, **31**, 120–5.

Held, T., Kummer, R., Marti, B. (1997) Heart rate, blood lactate concentration and subjective stress perception in submaximal running: New nomograms for assessment of endurance capacity. *Schweizerische Medizinische Wochenschrift*, **127**, 978–87.

Held, T., Marti, B. (1999) Substantial influence of level of endurance capacity on the association of perceived exertion with blood lactate accumulation. *International Journal of Sports Medicine*, **20**, 34–9.

Hetzler, R.K., Seip, R.L., Boutcher, S.H., Pierce, E., Snead, D., Weltman, A. (1991) Effect of exercise modality on ratings of perceived exertion at various lactate concentrations. *Medicine and Science in Sports and Exercise*, **23**, 88–92.

Hiatt, W.R. (1991) Exercise physiology in cardiovascular diseases. *Current Opinions in Cardiology*, **6**, 745–9.

Hill, D.W., Cureton, K.J., Grisham, S.C., Collins, M.A. (1987) Effect of training on the rating of perceived exertion at the ventilatory theshold. *European Journal of Applied Physiology*, **56**, 206–11.

Hoberg, E., Schuler, G., Kunze, B., Obermoser, A.L., Hauer, K., Mautner, H.P. (1990) Silent myocardial ischemia as a potential link between lack of premonitoring symptoms and increased risk of cardiac arrest during physical stress. *American Journal of Cardiology*, **65**, 583–9.

Hughson, R.L., Smyth, G.A. (1983) Slower adaptation of VO_2 to steady state of sub-maximal exercise with beta-blockade. *European Journal of Applied Physiology and Occupational Physiology*, **52**, 107–10.

Kang, J., Robertson, R.J., Goss, F.L., DaSilva, S.G., Visich, P., Suminski, R.R., *et al.* (1996) Effect of carbohydrate substrate availability on ratings of perceived exertion during prolonged exercise of moderate intensity. *Perceptual and Motor Skills*, **82**, 495–506.

Kang, J., Robertson, R.J., Goss, F.L., DaSilva, S.G., Suminski, R.R., Utter, A.C. (1997) Metabolic efficiency during arm and leg exercise at the same relative intensities. *Medicine and Science in Sports and Exercise*, **29**, 377–82.

Karageorghis, C.I., Terry, P.C. (1997) The psychophysical effects of music in sport and exercise: A review. *Journal of Sport Behaviour*, **20**, 54–68.

Karvonen, M.J., Kentala, F., Mustala, O. (1957) The effects of training on heart rate: A longitudinal study. *Annales Medicinae Experimentalis et Biologiae Fenniae*, **35**, 307–15.

Kohl, R.M., Shea, C.H. (1988) Perceived exertion: Influences of locus of control and expected work intensity and duration. *Journal of Human Movement Studies*, **15**, 225–72.

Krogh, A., Lindhard, J. (1920) The relative value of fat and carbohydrate as sources of muscular energy. *Biochemical Journal*, **14**, 290.

Lakomy, J., Lakomy, H.K.A. (1993) Estimation of maximum oxygen uptake from sub-maximal exercise on a Concept II rowing ergometer. *Journal of Sports Sciences*, **11**, 227–32.

Lamont, L.S., Romito, R.C., Finkelhor, R.S., Kalhan, S.C. (1997) Beta1-adrenoreceptors regulate resting metabolic rate. *Medicine and Science in Sports and Exercise*, **29**, 769–74.

Lavie, C.J., Milani, R.V. (2000) Disparate effects of improving aerobic exercise capac-ity and quality of life after cardiac rehabilitation in young and elderly coronary patients. *Journal of Cardiopulmonary Rehabilitation*, **20**, 235–40.

Liu, X., Brodie, D.A., Bundred, P.E. (2000) Difference in exercise heart rate, oxygen uptake and ratings of perceived exertion relationships in male post-myocardial infarction patients with and without beta blockade therapy. *Coronary Health Care*, **4**, 48–53.

Maass, U., Cachovan, M., Alexander, K. (1983) Effect of interval training on walking distance, hemodynamics and ventilation in patients with intermittent claudication: Changes of hemodynamics and ventilation. *Vasa*, **12**, 326–32.

Maresh, C., Noble, B.J. (1984) Utilization of perceived exertion ratings during exercise testing and training. In *Cardiac Rehabilitation: Exercise Testing and Prescription* (eds L.K. Hall, G.C. Meyer and H.K. Hellerstein), Spectrum, Great Neck, NY, pp. 155–73.

McArdle, W.D., Katch, F.I., Katch, V.L. (2001) *Exercise Physiology; Energy, Nutrition and Human Performance*, 5th edn, Williams and Wilkins, Baltimore, MD.

Meyer, K., Bucking, J. (2004) Exercise in heart failure: Should aqua therapy and swimming be allowed? *Medicine and Science in Sports and Exercise*, **36**, 2017–23.

Meyer, K., Lehmann, M., Sunder, G., Keul, J., Weidemann, H. (1990) Interval versus continuous exercise training after coronary bypass surgery: A comparison of train-ing-induced acute reactions with respect to the effectiveness of the exercise methods. *Clinical Cardiology*, **13**, 851–61.

Miles, D.S., Cox, M.H., Bomze, J.P. (1989) Cardiovascular responses to upper body exercise in normals and cardiac patients. *Medicine and Science in Sports and Exercise*, **21**, S126–31.

Morgan, W.P. (1973) Psychological factors influencing perceived exertion. *Medicine and Science in Sports and Exercise*, **5**, 97–103.

Morgan, W.P. (1994) Psychological components of effort sense. *Medicine and Science in Sports and Exercise*, **26**, 1071–7.

Morgan, W. (2000) Psychological factors associated with distance running and the marathon. In *Marathon Medicine* (ed. D. Tunstall-Pedoe), Royal Society of Medicine Press, London.

Moyna, N.M., Robertson, R.J., Meckes, C.L., Peoples, J.A., Millich, N.B., Thompson, P.D. (2001) Intermodal comparison of energy expenditure at exercise intensities corresponding to the perceptual preference range. *Medicine and Science in Sports Exercise*, **33**, 1404–10.

Myers, J., Froelicher, V.F. (1993) Exercise testing: Procedures and implementation. *Cardiology Clinics*, **11**, 199–213.

Neilsen, B., Rowell, L.B., Bonde-Petersen, F. (1984) Cardiovascular responses to heat stress and blood volume displacements during exercise in man. *European Journal of Applied Physiology*, **52**, 370–4.

Nethery, V.M. (2002) Comparison between internal and external sources of information during exercise: Influence on RPE and the impact of the exercise mode. *Journal of Sports Medicine and Physical Fitness*, **42**, 172–8.

Newsolme, E.A., Blomstrand, E., Ekblom, B. (1992) Physical and mental fatigue: Metabolic mechanisms and importance of plasma amino acids. *British Medical Bulletin*, **48**, 477–95.

Noble, B.J. (1982) Clinical applications of perceived exertion. *Medicine and Science in Sports and Exercise*, **14**, 406–11.

Noble, B., Robertson, R. (1996) *Perceived Exertion*. Human Kinetics, Champaign, IL.

Oldridge, N.B., Stoedefalke, K.G. (1984) Compliance and motivation in cardiac exercise programs. *Clinical Sports Medicine*, **3**, 443–54.

Omiya, K., Itoh, H., Harada, N., Maeda, T., Tajima, A., Oikawa, K., *et al.* (2004) Relationship between double product break point, lactate threshold, and ventilatory threshold in cardiac patients. *European Journal of Applied Physiology*, **91**, 224–9.

Parfitt, G., Eston, R. (1995) Changes in ratings of perceived exertion and psychological affect in the early stages of exercise. *Perceptual and Motor Skills*, **80**, 259–66.

Parfitt, G., Rose, E.A., Markland, D. (2000) The effect of prescribed and preferred intensity on psychological affect and the influence of baseline measures of affect. *Journal of Health Psychology*, **5**, 231–40.

Pearson, S.B., Banks, D.C., Patrick, J.M. (1979) The effect of beta-adrenoreceptor blockade on factors affecting exercise tolerance in normal man. *British Journal of Clinical Pharmacology*, **8**, 143–8.

Physiotools © (2005) Finland.

Pivarnik, J.M., Senay, L.C. (1986) Effect of endurance training and heat acclimation on perceived exertion during exercise. *Journal of Cardiopulmonary Rehabilitation*, **6**, 499–504.

Pokan, R., Hofmann, P., von, Duvillard, S.P., Beaufort, F., Smekal, G., Gasser, R., *et al.* (1998) The heart rate performance curve and left ventricular function during exercise in patients after myocardial infarction. *Medicine and Science in Sports and Exercise*, **30**, 1475–80.

Pollock, M.L., Wilmore, J.H., Fox, S.M. (1978) *Health and Fitness Through Physical Activity*, American College of Sports Medicine Series, John Wiley & Sons, New York.

Potteiger, J.A., Weber, S.F. (1994) Rating of perceived exertion and heart rate as indicators of exercise intensity in different environmental temperatures. *Medicine and Science in Sports and Exercise*, **26**, 791–6.

Poulsen, S.H. (2001) Clinical aspects of left ventricular diastolic function assessed by Doppler echocardiography following acute myocardial infarction. *Danish Medical Bulletin*, **48**, 199–210.

Prins, J., Cutner, D. (1999) Aquatic therapy in the rehabilitation of athletic injuries. *Clinical Sports Medicine*, **18**, 447–61, ix.

Reents, S. (2000). *Sport and Exercise Pharmacology*, Human Kinetics, Champaign, IL.

Rejeski, W.J. (1981) The perception of exertion: A social psychophysiological integration. *Journal of Sport Psychology*, **4**, 305–20.

Robertson, R.J., Noble, B.J. (1997) Perception of physical exertion: Methods, mediators and applications. *Exercise and Sports Science Reviews*, **25**, 407–52.

Robinson, S. (1938) Experimental studies of physical fitness in relation to age. *Arbeitphysiolgie*, **10**, 251.

Saltin, B., Boushel, R., Secher, N, Mitchell, J. (2000) *Exercise and Circulation in Health and Disease*, Human Kinetics, Champaign, IL.

Scottish Intercollegiate Guidelines Network (SIGN) (2002) *Cardiac Rehabilitation*, no. 57. Edinburgh.

Secher, N.H. (1993) Physiological and biomechanical aspects of rowing; Implications for training. *Sports Medicine*, **15**, 24–42.

Seip, R.L., Snead, D., Pierce, E.F., Stein, P., Weltman, A. (1991) Perceptual responses and blood lactate concentration: Effect of training state. *Medicine and Science in Sports and Exercise*, **23**, 80–7.

Singh, S.J., Morgan, M.C.D.L., Scott, S., Walters, D., Hardman, A.E. (1992) Development of a shuttle-walking test of disability in patients with chronic airways obstruction. *Thorax*, **47**, 1019–24.

Sjoberg, H., Frankenhaeuser, M., Bjurstedt, H. (1979) Interactions between heart rate, psychomotor performance and perceived effort during physical work as influenced by beta-andrenergic blockade. *Biological Psychology*, **8**, 31–43.

Skinner, J.S., Gaskill, S.E., Rankinen, T., Leon, A.S., Rao, D.C., Wilmore, J.H., *et al.* (2003) Heart rate vs % VO$_2$ max: Age sex, race, initial fitness and training response – HERITAGE study. *Medicine and Science in Sports and Exercise*, **35**, 1908–13.

Smutok, M.A., Skrinar, G.S., Pandolf, K.B. (1980) Exercise intensity: Subjective regulation by perceived exertion. *Archives of Physical Medicine and Rehabilitation*, **61**, 569–74.

Soenstrom, R.J. (1984) Exercise and self-esteem. *Exercise and Sport Science Reviews*, **12**, 123–55.

Song, K.J. (2003) The effects of self-efficacy promoting cardiac rehabilitation program on self-efficacy, health behavior, and quality of life. *Taehan Kanho Hakhoe Chi*, **33**, 510–18.

Stephens, T. (1988) Physical activity and mental health in the United States and Canada: Evidence from four population surveys. *Preventive Medicine*, **17**, 35–47.

Sukenik, S., Flusser, D., Abu-Shakra, M. (1999) The role of spa therapy in various rheumatic diseases. *Rheumatic Diseases Clinics of North America*, **25**, 883–97.

Sullivan, M.J., Higginbotham, M.B., Cobb, F.R. (1989) Exercise training in patients with chronic heart failure delays ventilatory anaerobic threshold and improves submaximal exercise performance. *Circulation*, **79**, 324–9.

Swain, D.P., Leutholtz, B.C. (1997) Heart rate reserve is equivalent to %VO_2 reserve, not to %VO_2max. *Medicine and Science in Sports and Exercise*, **29**, 410–14.

Swaine, I.L., Emmett, J., Murty, D., Dickinson, C., Dudfield, M. (1995) Rating of perceived exertion and heart rate relative to ventilatory threshold in women. *British Journal of Sports Medicine*, **29**, 57–60.

Sykes, K. (1995) Capacity assessment in the workplace: a new step test. *Journal of Occupational Health*, **1**, 20–2.

Sykes, K., Roberts, A. (2004) The Chester step test – a simple yet effective tool for the prediction of aerobic capacity. *Physiotherapy*, **90**, 183–8.

Tanaka, H., Monahan, K.D., Seals, D.R. (2001) Age-predicted maximal heart rate revisited. *Journal of the American College of Cardiology*, **37**, 153–6.

Thomas, T.R., Ziogas, G., Smith, T., Zhang, Q., Londeree, B.R. (1995) Physiological and perceived exertion responses to six modes of submaximal exercise. *Research Quarterly of Exercise and Sport*, **66**, 239–46.

Thow, M.K., McGregor, C., Rafferty, D. (2004) A study of the fitness levels of phase IV men, *European Journal of Cardiovascular Prevention and Rehabilitation*, **11**(1), 061.

Tobin, D., Thow, M.K. (1999) The 10m Shuttle Walk Test with Holter monitoring: An objective outcome measure for cardiac rehabilitation. *Coronary Health Care*, **3**, 3–17.

Todd, I.C., Wosornu, D., Stewart, I., Wild, T. (1992) Cardiac rehabilitation following myocardial infarction. A practical approach. *Sports Medicine*, **14**, 243–59.

Ueda, T., Kurokawa, T. (1995) Relationships between perceived exertion and physiological variables during swimming. *International Journal of Sports Medicine*, **16**, 385–9.

Utter, A., Kang, J., Nieman, D., Warren, B. (1997) Effect of carbohydrate substrate availability on ratings of perceived exertion during prolonged running. *International Journal of Sports Nutrition*, **7**, 274–85.

van Herwarden, C.L., Binkhorst, R.A., Fennis, J.F., van Laar, A. (1979) Effects of propanolol and metoprolol on haemodynamic and respiratory indices and on perceived exertion during exercise in hypertensive patients. *British Heart Journal*, **41**, 99–105.

Whaley, M.H., Brubaker, P.H., Kaminsky, L.A., Miller, C.R. (1997) Validity of rating of perceived exertion during graded exercise testing in apparently healthy adults and cardiac patients. *Journal of Cardiopulmonary Rehabilitation*, **17**, 261–7.

Wilcox, R.G., Bennett, T., MacDonald, I.A., Herbert, M., Skene, A.M. (1984) The effects of acute or chronic ingestion of propanolol or metoprolol on the physiological responses to prolonged, submaximal exercise in hypertensive men. *British Journal of Clinical Pharmacology*, **17**, 273–81.

Williams, J.G., Eston, R.G. (1989) Determination of the intensity dimension in vigorous exercise programmes with particular reference to the use of the rating of perceived exertion. *Sports Medicine*, **8**, 177–89.

Yates, B.C., Price-Fowlkes, T., Agrawal, S. (2003) Barriers and facilitators of self-reported physical activity in cardiac patients. *Research in Nursing and Health*, **26**, 459–69.

Zeni, A.I., Hoffman, M.D., Clifford, P.S. (1996) Energy expenditure with indoor exercise machines. *Journal of the American Medical Association*, **275**, 1424–7.

Chapter 4

Exercise Prescription in Cardiac Rehabilitation

Hilary Dingwall, Kim Ferrier and Joanne Semple

Chapter outline

The previous chapter explored the scientific dimension of exercise and monitoring. The next two chapters take the scientific principles and merge them with the art of exercise prescription and class design. An understanding of exercise physiology is necessary, but the experience, insight and creativity of the exercise prescriber is indispensable.

This chapter begins with an introduction to care, activity and exercise in phases I and II, addressing the skills and understanding required when working with patients in the early stages of recovery. The chapter then defines the principles for warm-up, overload and cool-down applicable to phases III and IV. The chapter expands on the **F**requency, **I**ntensity, **T**ime and **T**ype (FITT) principles for the overload period and for resistance training introduced in the previous chapter. A brief review of different methods which can be used to monitor exertion, including the rate of perceived exertion (RPE) scale (Borg, 1982) HR monitoring and metabolic values is provided. Finally, adaptations of the FITT principle for a variety of special considerations and co-pathologies that often complicate exercise prescription are included.

ACCUMULATED ACTIVITY AND STRUCTURED EXERCISE

The cardioprotective and psychosocial benefits require CR participants to engage in regular habitual exercise (SIGN, 2002). Exercise and activity should be integrated into all phases of CR. As there are different methods for prescribing activity and exercise, it is important to define the differences between physical activity and exercise in order to establish the impact both have on coronary heart disease.

Physical activity is described as bodily movement produced by skeletal muscles that requires energy expenditure and produces progressive healthy benefits, for example walking, housework, etc. (SIGN, 2002; ACSM 1998). **Exercise** is a type of physical activity that is planned, structured and repetitive, involving bodily movement performed to improve or maintain one or more components of physical fitness (Leon, NIH Consensus Statement, 1997). In 1997 the Health Education Board for Scotland (HEBS) devised a two-stage approach to encouraging the Scottish population to become more active. Many other national guidelines have adopted a similar approach.

Stage one

The first stage of the recommendation encourages realistic and achievable exercise prescription for the majority of the population. An active lifestyle does not require a structured exercise programme, but it encourages an increase in daily activity where activity is accumulated over a day (Pate, *et al.*, 1995). This proved a change in philosophy; previously the health message invoked a strenuous, more formal type of training. The message behind the first stage encourages moderate intensity exercise, accumulating 30 minutes or more per day on most, preferably all, days of the week (Pate, *et al.*, 1995). The activity can be accumulated in multiple small bouts of activity, for example three ten-minute bouts of walking.

Stage one targets adults who are currently inactive or who are not regularly active, and aims to encourage an accumulation of moderate intensity activity on most days of the week. This stage encourages active living, using the stairs instead of the escalator, walking the children to school instead of driving, etc. Despite the intensity being too low to gain significant improvements in aerobic fitness Franklin (1993), ACSM (2001) and Blair and Church (2004) have shown that activity at this lower intensity will offer substantial benefits across a broad range of health outcomes. These benefits include:

- improved bone density;
- improved glucose tolerance;
- reduced body fat;
- reduced total cholesterol and triglycerides;
- reduced risk of developing high blood pressure;
- psychosocial well being.

In addition, when subjects become more active by accumulated activity they may start to consider participation in more structured activity, as in stage two. All CR patient groups and sedentary individuals should be encouraged to be more active as well as take part in structured activity.

Stage two

The second stage targets adults who are already achieving stage one. In addition to the more active lifestyle in stage two, there is a need for these individuals to achieve exercise overload. The exercise prescription for these individuals must be at a higher intensity, with longer duration of continuous or intermittent activity. A frequency of three to five times per week is advocated for these patients (Pollock, *et al.*, 1998).

Exercise prescribers can motivate sedentary individuals to initiate and accumulate activity into their lifestyle by using stage one. By targeting patients who already engage in an active lifestyle, exercise prescribers can introduce new activities, integrate the FITT principles and encourage long-term adherence to exercise. Cardiac rehabilitation structured exercise classes will provide an ideal method to deliver exercise to these individuals. They may present with a variety of self-motivating and limiting factors and differing experiences of exercise. It is the role and responsibility of the exercise leader and CR team to work in partnership with the patient and family to prescribe and deliver a safe, effective and enjoyable experience of both activity and exercise.

PHASE I CARDIAC REHABILITATION

Phase I is the in-patient stage and includes medical evaluation, reassurance and education, correction of cardiac misconceptions, risk factor assessment, mobilisation and discharge planning SIGN (2002). Risk stratification should begin at this stage (see Chapter 2).

For patients post-MI, the site and size of the infarct can affect prognosis. Anterior infarcts often result in greater left ventricular dysfunction (BACR, 2000), and, as a consequence, exercise tolerance may be limited. Progression should vary according to the stability of the patient's condition during recovery, with higher risk or more debilitated patients progressing more slowly than lower risk, uncomplicated ones (AACVPR, 1999).

Previously, patients were often kept on bed rest for many weeks following a cardiac event. However, it is now recognised that prolonged period of immobilization can lead to deep vein thrombosis, pulmonary embolism, deconditioning, increased anxiety and depression (BACR, 1995). Over the years the period of bed rest and length of inpatient stay has gradually reduced. Patients post-MI are commonly allowed to sit up after a short period of bed rest, e.g. 12 to 24 hours (AACVPR, 1999). A prolonged period of bed rest may be required for patients who are haemodynamically unstable, or for those who have suffered shock, heart failure or serious arrhythmia.

Initial discussion about the patients' subjective description of their symptoms is important and patients should be encouraged to monitor for any adverse symptoms. Medical staff should be informed by the patient of any chest pain, shortness of breath, dizziness, palpitations or general ill health, and should be referred for further assessment. Initial activities should be monitored and the medical staff should have a good understanding of cardiac signs and symptoms. Activity should be introduced and gradually increased as soon as the patient is stable and pain free. This will vary according to the individual and the local protocol. Initial mobility is around the bedside and includes activities of daily living, such as washing and toileting. Circulatory exercises should be encouraged for all patient groups. Surgical patients may require breathing exercises including breathing control. If there are no adverse symptoms or post-surgical complications, a graduated walking programme is usually the method of choice. Within phase I, distance can be pre-set using marked distances in corridors within the ward. For example, one lap of the ward equals 50 yards. This can help to prescribe and monitor walking in phase I. Where appropriate, stair climbing should be introduced, and those requiring stair use at home should be able to climb stairs safely prior to discharge. Following CABG upper limb and neck mobility exercises should be carried out in order to maintain movement around the shoulder girdle and wound area. These exercises are required to prevent muscle shortening and adhesions developing (Pollock, *et al.*, 2000). Patients post-CABG can begin these exercises 24 hours after surgery (Pollock, *et al.*, 2000).

Pre-event mobility levels, age and other co-morbidities will also influence progression. It is important that progress is not only determined by local protocol, but that these factors and their clinical state are considered. Exercise tolerance should be monitored and activity increased as tolerated. However, activities should be restricted to 2–3 METs at this stage (BACR, 2000). The RPE (Borg, 1982) scale should be introduced at this stage with activity restricted to less than 13 RPE (ACSM, 2001). It is important to introduce as early as possible exercise/activity self-monitoring skills and to reinforce them during phase I (see Chapter 3). Ideally, the same staff member should see the patient throughout phase I to allow for a reliable assessment of exercise tolerance and to establish rapport.

Prior to discharge, an individualised exercise and activity plan should be prescribed for phase II. In addition, resumption of sexual activity, driving and returning to work should be discussed. It is important to identify any misconceptions and to discuss patient goals to ensure they are safe and realistic. An exercise consultation, prior to discharge, should be carried out in order to help the patient plan and adhere to phase II activity and exercise (see Chapter 8). Advice should be individualised, clear and concise, as patients often have difficulty absorbing information in hospital. This may be linked to feelings of anxiety and depression, which can be a natural reaction following a cardiac event (SIGN, 2002).

Similarly, family members are often frightened when their loved ones first go home, can be overprotective and limit activity. By involving family and friends in discussions, they too can be informed about appropriate levels of activity at phase II and receive the support they require. Social support from those at home is important and can improve prognosis by providing emotional support and sustaining activity and other healthy lifestyles (Yusuf, *et al.*, 2003).

PHASE II CARDIAC REHABILITATION

Phase II is the immediate post-discharge phase and normally lasts between 4 and 6 weeks. Often this period at home can be frightening for the patient and significant others. The family may feel isolated after being through a period of close supervision in the hospital environment. Despite these concerns, this phase of rehabilitation is often neglected (BACR, 2000).

Phase II is recognised as the stage where patients initiate some of the lifestyle changes and gradually begin to resume their normal daily activities. Support and guidance are normally provided by cardiac rehabilitation nurses, practice nurses and GPs, although other healthcare team members may also become involved, depending on patient need. This is commonly provided through telephone contact or home visits.

Use of the Heart Manual (Lewin, *et al.*, 1992) is commonly provided in this phase for patients post-MI. This six-week self-help rehabilitation programme is usually introduced by a facilitator during the in-patient phase and addresses health education, exercise and stress management.

Prior to discharge, an individualised activity plan should be prescribed for phase II. An incremental walking plan that is safe and realistic for the individual is often used. A gradual increase in time and distance and the inclusion of a warm-up and cool-down should be encouraged; however, at this stage the pace should be comfortable (BACR, 2000). Intensity should be restricted to less than 4 METS at this stage, frequency of walking should be daily with progression to 30 minutes continuous activity (BACR, 2000; ACSM, 2001). The RPE (Borg, 1982) scale should be used with activity restricted to less than 13 RPE (ACSM, 2001). A pedometer is a useful way for the patient and cardiac care team to monitor walking and progression. In addition, it can help to provide feedback and motivate the patient. Progress will vary but patients should be made aware of how they should feel, avoiding symptoms of over-activity and taught how to manage activity levels accordingly.

Many patients tire easily in the early stages, but this should gradually diminish (BHF, 2002). Safety considerations, including extreme weather conditions, exercise after food and alcohol, symptom management and glyceryl trinctrate (GTN) use should also be discussed (BACR, 2000).

Dusting, light cooking and other light household tasks should be encouraged initially. Other tasks, such as hoovering, should be left until the patient feels able, or at least until one to two weeks. Around the garden only light tasks are permitted, and this should be emphasised. Heavier tasks and do-it-yourself should be discussed at phase III. Return to sexual relationships should be discussed. Patients should be informed that when they can comfortably climb two flights of stairs they are safe to return to sexual relationships (BHF, 2001). However, post-CABG patients should wait for approximately four weeks (BHF, 2002). A comfortable position should be encouraged, and the partner may want to adopt the more active role initially.

PHASE III CARDIAC REHABILITATION

Phase III is traditionally the phase where structured exercise is the key element. The aim of phase III is to deliver safe and effective exercise. In addition, during this phase the aim is to help the patients learn to self-monitor their exercise and to increase safely activity at home and in other exercise environments.

Warm-up

The purpose of the warm-up is to prepare the muscular, nervous, cardiac, respiratory and vascular systems for the main workout. In other words, a warm-up prepares the body for the change from rest to exercise. The warm-up should be carried out at a low intensity and speed, repetition and exertion should be progressively increased. This graduated approach allows the heart to adapt to increased demand and to avoid the myocardial ischaemia and arrhythmias that may be provoked by sudden strenuous exercise (Dimsdale, *et al.*, 1984). Strenuous exercise without a warm-up can produce ischaemic ST segment changes and arrhythmias, even in healthy individuals (ACPICR, 2003). The warm-up should include: pulse-raising exercises, mobility exercises and preparatory stretches as follows:

PULSE-RAISING EXERCISES

These exercises gradually elevate the heart rate, thus giving the heart time to increase stroke volume and cardiac output. For patients with residual ischaemic/angina, a slow elevation will extend this threshold (BACR, 1995). During exercise, increased oxygen demands on the heart muscle are met through vasodilation of the coronary arteries, caused by local chemical changes (increase in CO_2 and lactic acid). In addition, the increase in myocardial oxygen requirement stimulates the sympathetic nervous system to release noradrenaline, causing further vasodilation of the coronary arteries. There is an associated increase in aortic pressure, which, due to the anatomy of the coronary arteries (situated at the bottom of the aorta), forces more blood into the coronary circulation. The ability of the body to maintain an adequate blood supply is important, as energy for the cardiac muscle relies almost entirely on aerobic metabolism. For those with residual ischaemia, this increase in oxygen supply will extend the threshold.

The warm-up should last for 15 minutes (BACR, 1995, ACSM, 2001), to allow for the necessary coronary adaptations to occur. The warm-up should gradually increase the heart rate to approximately 20 beats·min^{-1} below the target HR recommended for the individual (Fardy, *et al.*, 1998) no more than 11 on the Borg RPE (Borg, 1998).

During the warm-up, arm exercises should be introduced gradually. Arm exercises above the head must be introduced slowly, so as to avoid sudden increases in SBP and RPP, as discussed in Chapter 3. The increase is due to the smaller muscle mass of the upper body, compared to the larger muscle mass of the lower body (Schwade, *et al.*, 1977).

MOBILITY EXERCISES

Mobility exercises, e.g. shoulder rolls and knee bends should be gradually introduced, interspersed with pulse-raising exercises. The purpose of mobility exercises is to prepare specific joints and muscles that will be used during the main workout. Mobility exercises also provide an opportunity for skill rehearsal. Skill rehearsal introduces exercises that are used in the cardiovascular section of the class and are especially relevant for new patients in the group.

PREPARATORY STRETCHES

Including stretching during the warm-up is a controversial issue. At present, there is little scientific evidence to support preparatory stretches during the warm-up. A preparatory stretch component in most exercise classes is common, but there is sparse evidence to suggest that stretching is more effective than a good warm-up (Anderson O., 2000). However, there is evidence that relates muscle tightness to muscle injury (Stickler, *et al.*, 1990). Regular stretching will increase and improve flexibility, which in turn improves movement quality (Anderson B., 2000). Preparatory stretching aims to prepare the main muscle groups that will be used in the conditioning component. Cold muscle will have less blood flow and, therefore, it will be relatively inelastic and potentially at a higher risk of strain (Stickler, *et al.*, 1990).

Preparatory stretching should be static and held at the end of available range position, until there is a sensation of mild discomfort, but not pain (AACVPR, 1999). Although there is some debate on the frequency and duration of preparatory stretching, current recommendations are for a static stretch held for approximately 10 seconds with four repetitions of each muscle group (ACSM, 2001). If stretches are included, they should be interspersed with pulse-raising exercises in order to maintain an elevated heart rate and prevent venous pooling and a drop in BP.

OVERLOAD EXERCISE PRESCRIPTION PRINCIPLES

If correct exercise prescription is carried out, improvements can be made not only to cardio-respiratory fitness but also to general health, disease prevention and psychosocial well being (Buckley, *et al.*, 1999; SIGN, 2002). To achieve these improvements any exercise programme must work the body systems harder than they are normally accustomed to work. This process is known as overload and can be applied to any aspect of exercise, including cardiovascular fitness, strength and flexibility training (ACSM, 2001). The body responds to the exercise stimulus by adapting to the increased exercise load. For example, individuals who are sedentary can overload their systems by walking at a faster pace than normal. Individuals who have been more active for a period of time will require their activity overload to be set at a higher intensity and/or to work for longer periods.

Gradually, as the individual adjusts to the exercise, subsequent exercise will need to be increased in order to continue to achieve overload. This process is known as progressive overload, and it should continue until the individual's training goals are achieved. In order to achieve this overload, the exercise prescriber must consider the FITT (E) or FITT (A) principle. This principle describes the relationship between frequency, intensity, time and type of exercise, and it is an essential tool when prescribing effective exercise. Exercise prescription must be individualised to increase the likelihood of enjoyment (E) and/or adherence (A).

FITT (E) and (A) stand for the following:

F = FREQUENCY = number of days per week
I = INTENSITY = exertion required
T = TIME = minutes per day
T = TYPE = specific activity
(E) = ENJOYMENT
(A) = ADHERENCE

CARDIAC REHABILITATION PHASE III OVERLOAD

Frequency

Early studies into phase III cardiac rehabilitation (CR) programmes were based on exercise/education sessions that ran three days per week for eight weeks or longer (Jolliffe, *et al.*, 2004). Various studies have been carried out to determine the optimum frequency for cardiac rehabilitation programmes. There is still on-going debate around this topic, but recent literature has shown that two–three times per week, for a minimum of eight weeks, is sufficient to achieve physiological and psychosocial adaptations (SIGN, 2002). It should be emphasised that for patients to gain the optimum physiological and psychosocial benefits they will require prolonged exposure to exercise. Thus phase III should be considered as the minimum time for these changes to occur. The patients and significant others should be strongly encouraged to maintain exercise into phase IV.

How and where phase III programmes are delivered will vary, but they are commonly held in a hospital or, more recently, in the community. The common goal is to encourage life-long adherence to improving and maintaining the individual's exercise habits. By individualising exercise prescription and involving the patients in the exercise consultation process (see Chapter 8), they are more likely to enjoy (E) and adhere (A) on a long-term basis. Benefits to health and fitness can only be achieved if exercise levels are maintained.

Intensity

One of the aims of a cardiac rehabilitation programme is to improve cardiovascular fitness and functional capacity. How hard an individual works to achieve this improvement will be dependent on the individual's current exercise ability, motivation and choice of exercise. Current guidelines recommend that the benefits of a cardiac rehabilitation programme will be gained when exercise intensity is low-to-moderate and designed to suit a range of fitness levels (SIGN, 2002). Recommended intensity for cardiac patients is 60–75% HRmax or 40–60% HRRmax and 12–15 RPE. This will vary according to the risk stratification of the patient, determined during the individual's initial assessment (as described in Chapter 2) and the agreed goals of the patient. Individuals with diminished functional capacity, or who have been identified as a higher risk, should start at a lower intensity (60% HRmax), and progress as able, whereas fitter or lower risk individuals can often work between 65 and 75% HRmax.

Certain medications may alter this prescription. Beta-blockers reduce the sub-maximal and maximal HR, so this will have to be taken into account when developing individualised training zones (see Chapter 3).

Increasing intensity

Depending on the patient, progression of intensity should be guided by the goals of the patient, vocational needs and their risk stratification. When work rate is chosen to increase intensity this can be indicated when there is a noticeable decrease in both HR (>5 beats·min^{-1}) and RPE (≥1.5 RPE points) for a known workload. In addition, observation by the exercise leader of the patient, the ease or difficulty of performing the class can add to the decision to increase intensity.

Setting training zones

There are different methods to ascertain training heart rate, and this will be dependent on the information available to the prescriber. Chapter 3 covers in detail setting training zones (see Table 3.1, p. 54) including their strengths and weaknesses. The methods include the following:

- maximal heart rate or peak heart rate;
- Karvonen (Karvonen, et al., 1957) method/heart rate reserve;
- predicted maximal heart rate;
- rating of perceived exertion;
- metabolic equivalents.

As described above, there is a variety of methods for determining the correct exercise intensity a participant should aim to achieve. However, it is essential that the exercise instructors do not neglect their skills of observation. Continual assessment of quality of movement, excessive sweating or shortness of breath, skin colour and general fatigue are indicators for an individual to reduce intensity.

Time

The aerobic conditioning phase of a cardiac rehabilitation programme should last between 20 and 30 minutes (ACPICR, 1999; SIGN, 2002). This does not include the warm-up and cool-down. The CR participant should also be encouraged to be active and to accumulate activity in their everyday activities, as in stage one (Pate, *et al.*, 1995).

Type

There are different ways that the training activity can be delivered. These methods include steady state, circuit interval or free aerobic. The ACSM (1995) define group exercise type or mode, in terms of three classifications:

1. constant in nature, with little variation in effort, where HR can be kept within specific limits, e.g. cycling, rowing;
2. fluctuating involving skilful activities, e.g. cross country skiing;
3. varying with skill and intensity, fluctuating significantly, e.g. competitive sports.

For phase III CR type one and two would be those that achieve the training effects, but also introduce some aspects of motor skill. In addition type two reflects functional activity, where HR does not stay constant, for example, climbing stairs and housework.

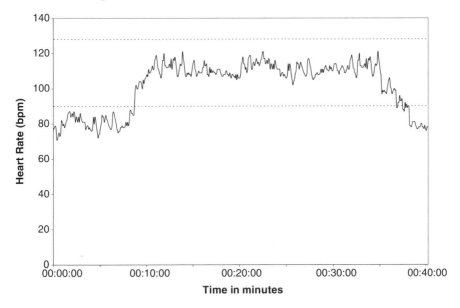

Figure 4.1. Heart rate pattern in a steady state exercise. Training heart rate zones between dotted lines.

Steady State Training

Steady state (like group one ACSM [1995]) training type is a sustained activity, where workload and HR are maintained at a constant sub-maximal intensity. Jogging, walking, stepping and cycling are examples of activities that are continuous. Figure 4.1 shows a steady state activity of cycling. The disadvantage of steady state training is that subjects can be bored. In addition, steady state does not represent normal functional activity, and is more difficult to transfer into a home environment.

Circuit Interval Training

In this context a circuit is a number of different exercise stations **NOT** circuit training. Circuit training involves a number of vigorous exercises that are often strength training in nature. Circuit interval training (like group two ACSM [1995]) involves short duration bursts of activity interspersed with either rest periods, or activity of a less intensive workload or active recovery (AR) stations. Cardiac rehabilitation phase III programmes tend to favour the use of circuit interval training as it allows for individualisation and accommodates different needs and levels of ability. This individualisation can be achieved through:

- changing the duration at each station;
- changing the length of rest periods between each station;
- altering the amount of resistance employed;
- altering the speed and range of movements.

When cardiac rehabilitation classes use circuit interval training, patients work between cardiovascular (CV) stations and active recovery (AR) stations. Each station has a fixed time period, which can range from 30 seconds to three minutes. CV stations should have the patients working up to the higher intensity of 75% HRmax, whereas AR are generally used to increase endurance of specific muscle groups, e.g. quadriceps, and are of a lower intensity, i.e. 60% HRmax. Patients exercise within the different HR and RPE ranges. The ultimate aim is to increase the duration of exercise at the higher intensity exercise stations and reduce the duration at the lower intensity stations. This is achieved by encouraging an increase in the duration of the CV component and a reduction in AR time. To attain overload, an increase in CV time or an increase in exercise intensity can be used. It will depend on the patient whether time or intensity is the more appropriate method to attain increase in overload.

This example shows how progression on a circuit with 5 CV and 5 AR stations can be achieved by increasing time spent at each station:

CIRCUIT ONE (10 MINUTES)
AR – 1 minute
CV – 1 minute
Total CV time = 5 minutes
Total AR time = 5 minutes

Progresses to:

CIRCUIT TWO (10 MINUTES)
AR – 30 seconds
CV – 1 minute, 30 seconds
Total CV time = 7.5 minutes
Total AR time = 2.5 minutes

Progresses to:

CIRCUIT THREE (USING 5 CV STATIONS ONLY)
AR – 0 minute
CV – 2 minutes
Total CV time = 10 minutes
Total AR time = 0 minutes

In this type of exercise the HR fluctuates and monitoring is more difficult. The advantage of this mode is that it is more representative of daily functional activity. In addition, it is easier for the exercise leader to construct a home

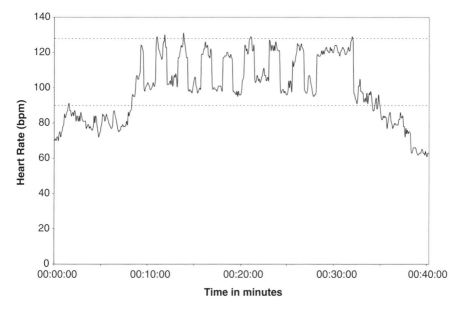

Figure 4.2. Heart rate pattern in an interval circuit exercise. Training heart rate zones between dotted lines.

programme that is similar to this. Figure 4.2 shows HR during circuit interval mode.

FREE AEROBIC

This type of training involves the exercise leader performing the exercise at the same time as the group and teaching the group at the same time. The class follows the exercise leader's commands and demonstrations. This type of activity is often used in the warm-up part of the class. Free aerobics can provide a large variety of exercises and require very little equipment. A disadvantage is that monitoring and maintaining subjects in their training zones are more difficult. (See Chapter 5 for more on class design.)

RESISTANCE TRAINING

Muscle strength, endurance and aerobic function are required for a fully active lifestyle (Pollock, *et al.*, 2000). Muscle strength is defined as the ability of a muscle or muscle group to produce maximal force at a given velocity of movement. Muscle endurance is the ability of a muscle or muscle group to perform repeated muscle actions against a sub-maximal resistance (ACSM, 2001).

Resistance exercise (RE) incorporates all types of strength and weight training and will lead to improvements in both muscle strength and endurance. RE has many proven health benefits, including increases in lean muscular mass, and it has been shown to complement aerobic exercise in the maintenance of basal metabolic rate, important for weight management (Pollock, *et al.*, 2000). In addition, RE can reduce the risk of falling by improving muscular strength and balance (ACSM, 2001). Favourable effects on bone density are associated with resistance exercise (Bjarnason-Wehrens, *et al.*, 2004). Many women in CR, if they are older, will be post-menopausal, and for this group prevention and treatment of osteoporosis are added benefits.

Many activities of daily living and occupational tasks require an equal amount, if not more, of upper body strength than aerobic fitness (Lindsay and Gaw, 1997). After a cardiac event people are often afraid to lift or to attempt resistance-based activities. Therefore, including supervised RE within a cardiac rehabilitation programme may help to resolve anxieties by providing advice on technique and prescription.

The incidence of coronary heart disease increases with age and after the menopause (BHFS, 2004). This coincides with an age-related decline in muscular strength and fat-free mass after the age of 50 (ACSM, 2001). RE has been shown to prevent decline in muscle strength and has shown favourable improvements in lean muscle mass (Pollock, *et al.*, 1998). These benefits support the inclusion of RE within a comprehensive cardiac rehabilitation programme.

Traditionally, cardiac rehabilitation focused on aerobic exercise due to concerns that BP increases during RE would increase cardiovascular complications. However, AACVPR (1999), the ACSM (2001) and SIGN (2002) now recommend RE as part of a comprehensive rehabilitation programme. With appropriate screening and supervision, fewer cardiovascular complications have been associated with RE than with aerobic endurance exercise (Bjarnason-Wehrens, *et al.*, 2004).

Most research on RE in the CR setting has been carried out on men with low to moderate cardiac risk. There is sparse evidence on the effects of RE on the higher-risk patient groups or on women. Previous studies suggested that the isometric component caused reduced ejection fraction, left ventricle wall motion abnormalities and increased incidence of arrhythmias (BACR, 2000). However, due to the lack of evidence, there is reluctance to include RE in the cardiac rehabilitation setting for high-risk patient groups (Pollock, *et al.*, 2000).

Contraindications to resistance

Contraindications to resistance exercise are similar to those for the aerobic component. For RE these include:

- abnormal haemodynamic responses with exercise;
- significant ischaemic changes during graded exercise testing;

- poor left ventricular function;
- uncontrolled hypertension or arrhythmias;
- exercise capacity <6 METs.

(BACR, 2000; ACPICR, 2003).

When to start resistance exercise

There is some dispute as to when coronary heart disease patients should commence an RE programme. There is general consensus that patients should complete a period of aerobic exercise prior to initiating resistance training. The ACSM (2001) and SIGN (2002) recommend a period of four to six weeks' aerobic acclimatisation. This period allows for patients' haemodynamic responses to exercise to be assessed and for any complications to be ruled out before progression to RE. Additionally, the patient can use this time to become familiar with self-monitoring and to establish the correct training intensity.

The ACSM (2001) suggest that patients post-MI and CABG should wait for four to six weeks post-event before commencing RE. For patients following percutaneus transluminal coronary angioplasty (PTCA) a shorter period of one to two weeks may be adequate (ACSM, 2001).

Prior to commencing upper limb resistance training CABG patients should have their wound and sternal area assessed, to ensure adequate healing and stability (Pollock, *et al.*, 2000). Caution is advised for patients who demonstrate symptoms of chest clicking or discomfort, as this can signify problems with healing. There is some evidence that an exercise programme should avoid any exercises that place strain on the sternal area for three months post-operation (Pollock, *et al.*, 2000). This will vary considerably between individuals, due to differences in pain tolerance and wound healing.

Exercise prescription for resistance training

Recommendations on the prescription of resistance training will be considered under the FITT principle.

FREQUENCY

To achieve the benefits of resistance training, a frequency of two to three days a week is recommended (AHA, 1995; AACVPR, 1999; SIGN, 2002). Training and rest days should be alternated to allow for muscle recuperation.

INTENSITY

Cardiac patients should start resistance training at a low intensity and slowly progress. Initially, the exercises may be taught with little or no resistance, in order to familiarise patients with safe technique. During RE the correct breathing pattern should be taught, in order to avoid the valsalva manoeuvre, when an individual forces exhalation against a closed glottis. During this manoeuvre there is an alteration in BP response, due to increased total peripheral resistance and reduced blood flow to muscles. The intrathoracic pressure increases, and this can reduce venous return and stroke volume. The result of these changes is increased myocardial oxygen demand when cardiac output is reduced (ACSM, 2001). To avoid valsalva, participants should be taught to breathe out during the contraction phase of the exercise and to breathe in during the relaxation phase (Fardy, *et al.*, 1998). They should also be taught why correct breathing is important and to breathe properly when carrying out daily activities that require moving or lifting loads.

In order to determine the correct workload, much of the literature refers to the one repetition maximum method (1RM), or maximum voluntary contraction. One RM is defined as the maximum weight that can be lifted in a smooth continuous movement, using proper technique without strain or breath-holding (Daub, *et al.*, 1996). An initial intensity that corresponds to 30–50% repetition maximum (RM) is recommended (AACVPR, 1999). A gradual increase in intensity is encouraged. However, most studies are based on low-risk cardiac patients using maximal workloads of 60–70% RPM (SIGN, 2002). High intensity levels may increase cardiovascular complications (Fardy, *et al.*, 1998). This maximal testing method for cardiac patients is controversial, due to the increased risk of valsalva and other cardiovascular complications (Bjarnason-Wehrens, *et al.*, 2004).

Others recommend a graded approach to resistance training (AACVPR, 1999; ACSM, 2001). Initially, the individual performs eight to ten repetitions using a lighter resistance and is closely monitored. When the patient can perform 12 to 15 repetitions without complications and with a good technique, the resistance is gradually increased. When using this method patients should be experiencing fatigue as they perform the last few repetitions. Table 4.1 shows load relationships for resistance training.

MONITORING RESISTANCE TRAINING

In order to monitor and guide the patient during RE, heart rate and Borg (1998) are the easiest to carry out in the cardiac rehabilitation setting. Heart rate may provide an appropriate guide to the patient during RE, as this method is often familiar to them. Heart rate should not exceed the maximum training intensity determined for the aerobic component. Heart rate response to RE is often lower than during the aerobic component and may not truly reflect the stress on the cardiovascular system.

The rate pressure produce (RPP) is higher during maximal isometric and dynamic resistance exercise than during maximal aerobic exercise, primarily because of a lower peak HR response (Pollock *et al.*, 2000). The elevation in

Table 4.1. Load repetition relationship for resistance training

% 1RM	Number of repetitions possible
60%	17
65%	14
70%	12
75%	10
80%	8
85%	6
90%	5
95%	3
100%	1

systolic blood pressure (SBP) contributes more than HR to the increase in RPP seen with RE (Fardy, *et al.*, 1998). When prescribing RE the instructor must consider the BP response, as HR alone will not truly reflect RPP, and, thus, what the patient can safely manage.

AACVPR (1999) recommends blood pressure monitoring during RE, but this can be difficult in the clinical setting. BP measurement at rest and recovery will not reflect changes during RE, as BP returns to normal quickly with rest (Bjarnason-Wehrens, *et al.*, 2004). Pollock, *et al.* (2000) suggest placing the BP cuff on the non-exercising limb. In a clinical environment safety is paramount. Therefore, due to these monitoring difficulties hypertensive patients should abstain from resistance exercise until their BP is controlled.

For those able to monitor heart rate and blood pressure during RE the RPP value can be calculated. The RPP value can be used as an effective method to monitor the patient and prescribe exercise. The patient should avoid exercise that evokes an RPP that produces significant ischaemia as seen during exercise testing. The RPP is usually calculated and displayed on exercise testing results. When these measurements cannot be accurately taken it is essential to monitor these patients closely during RE training.

The Borg (1998) scale is often considered a more useful tool during RE. The patient should not experience greater exertion during RE than in the aerobic component. On the 6 to 20 Borg (1998) point scale participants should be advised to work between 11 to 14 'fairly light' to 'somewhat hard' (ACSM, 2001). Regardless of the method used, the patients' response to RE should be closely monitored. Any symptoms of abnormal shortness of breath, chest pain, dizziness or irregular heart rhythm problems are contra-indicative, and exercise should be stopped immediately (ACSM, 2001).

TIME

The resistance component should last between 20 and 30 minutes and should be performed after the aerobic component (Fardy, *et al.*, 1998), as it will ensure adequate warm-up prior to RE. Rest periods between each exercise and each set should be relatively short in order to maximise benefits (ACSM, 2001). Any time between 15 seconds and one minute is advised. Longer rest periods will reduce the endurance benefits. However, if safety is the main concern HR and BP will recover if the rest periods consist of one minute or more (Fardy, *et al.*, 1998).

TYPE

There are two main types of muscular contraction: isotonic and isometric. An isotonic contraction produces a dynamic movement and imposes a volume load to the left ventricle. An isometric contraction is a static muscular contraction without movement, e.g. handgrip which imposes a pressure load to the left ventricle. Blood flow does not increase to the non-contracting muscles during isometric exercise because of reflex vasoconstriction. The combination of vasoconstriction and increased cardiac output during isometric contraction causes a disproportionate rise in systolic, diastolic and mean blood pressure (Pollock, *et al.*, 2000).

BP response has a direct effect on the RPP and myocardial workload, and a high BP response will increase the risk of myocardial ischaemia. To minimise this increased BP response, isotonic work or dynamic resistance training is recommended for the cardiac population. A further benefit of this type of exercise is that it reflects normal activities of daily living.

The blood pressure and HR response during RE are also proportional to the size of the muscle mass involved (Meyer, 2001). Thus, any RE targeting both upper limbs simultaneously will result in a greater response than single-limb exercise. Therefore, the extent of muscle mass involved will have a direct effect on the RPP. To prevent a large increase in the RPP value and to minimise myocardial ischaemia, the exercise prescriber must consider muscle mass and adapt exercise appropriately. This is particularly important for patients who demonstrate an exaggerated BP response during RE or significant ischaemia at a given RPP. For this group, single-limb exercises should be used rather than double-limb (ACSM, 2001).

All exercises should be rhythmical in nature, moving through a full range of movement and performed at a moderate to slow controlled speed. The exercise leader and assistants should observe the quality of RE task performed by the patient. Weights should be moved in a slow, sustained, controlled manner with exhalation during the straining part of the lift (ACSM, 2001).

The programme should include eight to ten exercises targeting different muscle groups (ACSM, 2001). The resistance exercises should target all major muscle groups to allow for all-round body conditioning: chest, back, biceps, triceps, abdominals, lower back, quadriceps, hamstrings and calves. The ACSM (2001) recommends exercising large muscle groups before small muscle groups. In an RE programme, exercises should alternate between upper and lower body work. This will give each muscle group recovery time (Fardy, *et al.*, 1998).

The number of sets of resistance exercise required for CR patients remains controversial. The AACVPR (1999) recommend one set of each exercise. Pollock, *et al.* (2000) suggest that strength gains are small with further sets. Additional sets would increase the total duration of the RE session, and this could reduce exercise adherence (ACPICR, 2003). Individuals may also be more at risk of rushing to complete exercises, which may detract from technique and increase the risk of injury. However, as seen in the overload section, further sets may be used as a method of progression to achieve overload (ACSM, 2001).

Resistance equipment

The type of exercise will depend on both the equipment and space available. Resistance bands and dumbbells are easily accessible and allow for a gradual progression in resistance or weight. Method of delivery can be either circuit-type group sessions or delivered by the exercise leader where the class performs the same exercise. Caution should be used for those with balance or grip problems who may drop weights.

RE can be performed using exercise mats on the floor. All floor exercises should be carried out together, as interspersing standing and floor exercises can increase the risk of venous pooling. This may also cause a sudden increase in preload and end diastolic volume which may lead to angina and arrhythmias (ACSM, 2001). Some patients may have difficulty getting up and down from the floor, which may have implications for the rest period between each circuit. Additionally, there may be a risk of orthostatic hypotension when returning to an upright posture (ACSM, 2001).

The use of multi-gym weight training is widely recommended, but can be an expensive option. Weight machines maintain equilibrium, ensure the movement plane is well controlled and have easily altered resistance. This mode of resistance training may be useful for those with balance difficulties because the machines provide support.

Prior to participating in RE patients should have an induction session. This is important to ensure safety. The induction should include advice and demonstration on positioning, moving and handling, and setting the resistance at the prescribed level. During all types of resistance training patients should be advised to avoid excess gripping and breath holding to help prevent valsalva. This advice should also be discussed in relation to heavy household or lifting tasks that are carried out at home or elsewhere.

Providing overload

As the individual progresses, the exercise dose should be increased in order to achieve overload as in the aerobic component. Overload will allow an increase in muscular strength and endurance and should be carried out over time. This can be achieved by:

- increasing the resistance or weight;
- increasing the repetitions;
- increasing the sets;
- decreasing the rest period between sets or exercises.

(ACSM, 2001).

To achieve overload, an initial increase in the number of repetitions is recommended before an increase in resistance (Fardy, *et al.*, 1998). When the patient can safely achieve 15 repetitions, the resistance should be gradually increased. Pollock, *et al.* (2000) recommend that resistance is increased by 2 to 5 lbs for the upper limbs and by 5 to 10 lbs for lower limbs. This will depend on training adaptations and the individual's progress. In order to elicit an increase in strength, more resistance, with fewer repetitions, is required. In order to elicit an increase in endurance, more repetitions of a low to moderate resistance are required (ACSM, 2001).

Exercise prescription and its progression should also take into account the needs of the individual. RE programmes should accommodate the daily living and occupational requirements of participants. Emphasis should be placed on specific muscles that individuals require for their occupation and activities, e.g. upper limb strength for building trade employment. In addition, return to domestic activities after a period of inactivity should be considered. Different occupations and lifestyles may require a varying amount of either strength or endurance. This should be taken into consideration when designing RE programmes.

The benefits seen in muscle mass and strength diminish when RE is stopped (ACSM, 2001). Therefore, it is important to encourage participants to maintain exercise, both aerobic and RE, at phase III and into phase IV.

COOL-DOWN

The cool-down should consist of pulse-lowering exercises, which aim to reduce the heart rate and blood pressure gradually. The time period recommended by SIGN (2002) for a cool-down session is 10 minutes and should consist of exercises of steadily diminishing intensity. Cool-down exercises should predominantly involve large muscle groups. Arm exercises should be kept to minimum and below shoulder height, to avoid increases in SBP and therefore RPP.

The cool-down component is the reverse of the warm-up component. A gradual reduction in intensity allows the muscular pumping action against the veins to assist venous return. This will prevent venous pooling, which can occur if exercise is stopped suddenly (ACSM, 2001).

Post-exercise hypotension is more common in cardiac patients as a result of the side effects of certain cardiac medications, and also due to the age-related slower reaction of the baroreceptors that detect changes in BP. In addition, after high-intensity exercise there is a risk of arrhythmias, due to the increased sympathetic activity (ACSM, 1995). A gradual cool-down will reduce the likelihood of these occurring.

Cool-down stretches

The aim of post-workout stretches is to maintain range of movement, and, if required, to improve flexibility of specific muscles (ACSM, 2001). Poor range of movement can lead to poor posture, injuries and fatigue; therefore, it is important to include these stretches at the end of the exercise session. One example of where this may be especially important is in post-CABG patients. This group may adopt poor posture as a consequence of sternal wound pain (Pollock, *et al.*, 2000). Stretching is particularly important to reduce adaptive shortening of the pectoral muscles and to maintain thoracic/upper body mobility.

Developmental stretches should be held for between 15 and 30 seconds with four repetitions of each muscle group (ACSM, 2000; Anderson, B, 2000). The patients should be encouraged to breathe normally, ease into the stretch and not to bounce. The stretch should be taken to a point of slight discomfort, but not pain. The exercise leader and assistants should be observing participants' performance for position and quality of the exercise and should correct poor technique.

Water-based Activities

Unfortunately, limited data are available on the actual energy cost of most water-based activities, especially in cardiac patients (Fardy, *et al.*, 1998). Participants can use a variety of swimming strokes, but may need to take care, especially following CABG surgery. Since swimming requires substantial use of the upper limbs, care must be taken to avoid excessive strain on the sternal bone, which may cause discomfort or aggravate existing wound pain. Participants may also need to modify their technique to ensure exercise prescription is adhered to. Most data regarding the energy requirements of swimming strokes are based on competitive swimmers and may not be relevant for cardiac patients (McArdle, *et al.*, 1991).

Of all the strokes, backstroke and breaststroke can be most easily modified to ensure the training intensity for each individual is attained. Conversely, the energy cost of front crawl can vary enormously, depending on the technique used (Fardy, *et al.*, 1998). Boone and Thompson (1983) and Fletcher, *et al.* (1984) advise that patients with cardiac disease not use front crawl. The front crawl may achieve an intensity level of 80–85% of HRmax, which is a higher intensity than the recommended 60–75% HRmax for cardiac patients.

Aqua-fit exercise, aerobic exercise performed in water, can be an alternative way to exercise in water. This can be a good method for patients with lower limb arthritis and for obese subjects. The same issues of water-based activity apply to aqua-fit. Other issues that need to be considered when prescribing water-based activities are:

POSITION

The positions swimmers adopt have an effect on the myocardial workload. The horizontal position one adopts when swimming will increase the return of blood to the heart. This in turn will increase preload (the tension exerted on the heart wall at the end of the diastolic phase), and it will also increase the force of the subsequent contraction. Increases in preload and in the force of contraction are two of the physiological parameters necessary to determine myocardial O_2 uptake (MVO_2). Therefore, swimming will increase the heart muscle's demand for oxygen.

CAPABILITY

The individual's capability must be taken into consideration prior to prescribing swimming as an exercise modality. By using HR or MET data from the results of the patients ETT or SWT the prescriber can assess whether swimming is an appropriate activity for their client. MET value tables generally view swimming between 8 to 10 METS. Swimming may be an inappropriate exercise if this level of activity has not been achieved in most recent fitness tests. Breaststroke is estimated at 8 to10 METS and the front crawl at 9 to 10 METS (ACPICR, 2003).

TEMPERATURE

The recommended pool temperature is between 26 and 33°C (89–92°F) (Koszota, 1989). Lower temperatures will allow for heat dissipation during exercise, but patients with joint problems or peripheral vascular disease (PVD) may prefer and benefit from warmer water. There are no studies on cardiac patients with chronic obstructive pulmonary disease (COPD) and their response to pool temperature. However, COPD clients may dislike being submerged to chest height, due to the baropressure exerted by the water; this may decrease chest expansion and lead to breathing difficulties. As discussed in Chapter 3 RPE is altered in water activity. RPE is not invalid during water-based activity, but it requires the target RPE to be about two points lower in water, compared to land-based exercise. (See Chapter 3 for more on physiological responses in water.)

PHASE IV

Before a patient moves from the phase III CR there should be strategies in place to help the patient graduate to phase IV. In addition, there should be good communication between phases III and IV, regarding changes in the medical or exercise status of the class members (see Chapter 6).

Exercise prescription in phase IV

Phase IV exercise should see a maintenance of individualised exercise using the same FITT principles as in previous phases. Participants graduating to phase IV after phase III should be more independent exercisers and more responsible for self-monitoring. During an exercise consultation, the phase IV participant may wish to try different activities, for example dancing, hill walking, etc. The exercise consultant should help participants select activity and exercise that will help maintain their health, interest and fitness.

PATIENT GROUPS WITH SPECIAL CONSIDERATIONS

Coronary heart disease tends to be an age-related condition. The statistics on CHD show that the rate of deaths caused by coronary heart disease increases with age, and especially in women post-menopause.

Age and coronary heart disease

The majority of patients presenting with CHD are aged 50 years and older. Figure 4.3 highlights the percentage of deaths from coronary heart disease recorded in the UK in 2002. As can be seen, there are higher numbers in the older age range.

Older patients often present with other co-pathologies (Thow, *et al.*, 2003). For the exercise prescriber, this poses a challenge to accommodate these other conditions while ensuring that the patient can exercise safely and without aggravating other pathologies.

The following section considers changes associated with ageing and co-pathologies often associated with the older patient and the CHD process. Where appropriate adaptations of the FITT principles for each are considered for the ageing process, hypertension, hypotension, obesity, diabetes, peripheral vascular disease, osteoarthritis and rheumatoid arthritis, and osteoporosis.

Ageing processes

As many individuals in the cardiac rehabilitation population are 50+ years of age, it is important that the exercise prescriber takes into account the

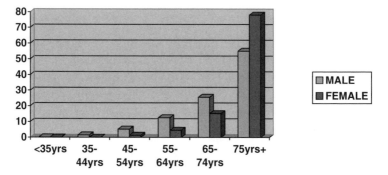

Figure 4.3. Deaths from coronary heart disease (BHF, CHD Statistics, 2002).

changes that are associated with ageing and the effect these will have on exercise.

CARDIOVASCULAR FUNCTION

There is loss of VO_2max by about 1% per year between the ages of 25 and 75 years (Shvartz and Reibold, 1990). This loss of functional capacity is not inevitable and appears to be closely related to reduced activity levels. The elasticity of the major blood vessels declines with age, resulting in an increase in both systolic and diastolic blood pressure. This increases peripheral resistance and in turn increases afterload (see Chapter 3), which can result in ventricular hypertrophy.

HEART RATE

Maximal HR will decline with age. This is thought to be due to a decrease in myocardial sensitivity to catecholamines and the effect of prolonged diastolic filling (ACSM, 2001). The predictive age-adjusted HR formula (see Chapter 3) does take this into consideration. Some care is required in using this formula, due to the limitation of over- or under-prescription. RPE may be more useful.

PULMONARY FUNCTION

Lung elasticity and chest cavity expansion decrease with age. Many older adults will increase their rate of breathing, rather than depth, to increase ventilation. This may result in additional work for the respiratory muscles, and many will describe symptoms of breathing discomfort during exercise. Advice on breathing control should be included where appropriate.

BONE

Women begin to lose bone at age 30, and will lose about 20% by the age of 65 and 30% by the age of 80. Men at the age of 40 onwards will lose 10 to 15% by the age of 70 and 20% by the age of 80 (ACSM, 2001). (See p. 128 on osteoporosis for exercise implications.)

STRENGTH

Muscle function decreases approximately 25% by the age of 65 (ACSM, 2001). This decline in strength generally begins at the age of 30 and will be more marked in women than men, and will be greater in the lower limbs than the upper limbs (BACR, 2000). Therefore it is appropriate to include RE in a comprehensive exercise programme.

JOINTS AND FLEXIBILITY

Both flexibility and range of movement will decline with age. Combined with reductions in strength, this may result in an increase likelihood of falls and may exacerbate arthritic problems. Incorporating flexibility exercises into the programme will help to reduce this risk.

BODY COMPOSITION

There will be a reduction in lean body mass and an increase in body fat (American Council on Exercise, 1998). Both men and women will gain weight, and this is generally a result of an imbalance of calorie intake and energy expenditure. Changes in metabolism will also contribute to weight gain. The increased energy expenditure associated with exercise and improved muscle/fat ratio will assist weight management (Pollock, *et al.*, 2000).

MOTOR SKILLS

Balance, reaction times and motor coordination deteriorate with age. When combined with deterioration in hearing and eyesight, these changes have been shown to increase the likelihood of falls by 35 to 40% in adults over 60 (ACSM, 2001). Participants may have difficulty hearing/seeing instructions, and this can lead to anxiety or loss of confidence. The exercise leader must consider the class environment in order to be sensitive to the specific needs of the participants. Although age deteriorates motor skills, it is important to incorporate them into CR exercise programmes to ensure practice and skill rehearsal. Balance and motor skills require practice.

Exercise for older people

FREQUENCY

For older adults there should be three to five structured sessions per week, and an active living approach should be encouraged, integrating activity into everyday life.

INTENSITY

For older adults intensity should be between 60 and 75% HRmax.

TYPE

Aerobic endurance, RE, flexibility, weight-bearing activities, motor skills and balance activities should be included.

TIME

Exercise should include as much functional accumulated activity as possible most days per week. The overload period should last for 20 to 30 minutes.

Hypertension

FREQUENCY

The frequency remains at 3–5 sessions per week, integrating activity into everyday life.

INTENSITY

The intensity should be reduced to 50 to 75% HRmax. SBP increases in proportion to the intensity of the activity. Moderate intensity activity should be prescribed to avoid large increases in SBP. When HR and SBP are elevated, the myocardium is working harder and requires more oxygen due to a large increase in RPP. Hypertensive patients have a higher resting BP and when coupled with the associated increase in SBP during exercise the RPP value will be higher. Therefore, higher intensity exercise should be avoided until hypertension is controlled.

TYPE

Aerobic activities should be prescribed with the following considerations: it is important that all exercises are dynamic, as isometric exercise will increase BP. Isometric activities associated with the valsalva manoeuvre should be avoided. Resistance training should be prescribed using lower resistance and higher repetitions, ensuring the patients are not over-gripping equipment.

When prescribing exercise for hypertensive patients it is important to remember the physiological response of SBP when exercising a smaller muscle mass, i.e. arms versus legs. A smaller muscle mass in the upper body will result in less vasodilation and an increase in total resistance to blood flow. When exercising the upper limbs, there will be a greater BP increase, when compared to exercise of the lower limbs. This difference in SBP response to the use of the arms versus legs has important implications for myocardial oxygen consumption. The BP increase with upper limbs will increase the RPP. Upper body exercise will require a higher myocardial oxygen demand and therefore less activity can be performed prior to the onset of ischaemia. Care should be taken when including upper limb activities in a hypertensive participant's exercise regime.

TIME

Gradually increase duration prior to increasing intensity, as shown for a circuit design (see Chapter 5).

Hypotension

SBP should increase with exercise. If there is a drop in BP during exercise, this is a very serious concern and a contraindication to exercise. A reduction in BP during graded exercise places patients at a higher risk for a cardiac event (Squires, 1998). During an exercise class patients should be advised to keep their feet moving at all times. This should include periods when patients may be having a rest, to avoid postural and orthostatic hypotension. An inadequate warm-up, cool-down or a sudden stop results in pooling of the blood in the lower extremities, i.e. reduced venous return. This will cause a drop in BP. Any sudden drop in BP from the individual's normal range may produce dizziness or lightheadedness.

A drop in BP can also be caused by some medications, e.g. beta-blockers, nitrates, ACE inhibitors and calcium channel blockers. Exercise prescribers and CR participants must be aware of the actions and implications for exercise of these medications. It is important that patients inform the instructor of the use of their GTN spray or any changes in medication.

Exercises where patients move from lying to standing should be avoided, as this may induce sudden changes in BP, which can lead to postural hypotension. This should be taken into account when designing a circuit. The other FITT principles should be applied as for a post-MI patient.

Obesity

Obesity is excess body fat for a given age or gender and can increase the risk of coronary heart disease two-fold (BHF, 2004). Body Mass Index (BMI) is an accepted method of estimating a person's relative weight. BMI is calculated by dividing weight in kilograms by the square of height in metres. The following are the differing ranges of BMI:

BMI 20–24.9 kg/m^2 = healthy, stable, weight range
BMI 25–29.9 kg/m^2 = overweight
BMI 30–39.9 kg/m^2 = obese
BMI 40 kg/m^2 and above = severely obese

(BACR, 2000).

In the last ten years the percentage of obese adults has increased by more than 50%, from 14% of the population to 22% (BHF, 2004). This has many serious implications for cardiac rehabilitation, as obesity is a significant risk to the primary cause and secondary prevention of CHD.

The management of weight loss is a controversial area. At present there is inconclusive evidence regarding the relative effectiveness of physical activity combined with diet, versus diet alone or physical activity alone (Mulvihill and Quigley, 2003). As adipose tissue contains about 7000 kcal/kg, with physical activity alone it is difficult to lose much weight (BHF, 2004). Therefore, management of obese participants should include advice on diet, physical activity and a behavioural modification component in order to be comprehensive and effective. The most favourable alterations in body composition will occur with low-intensity, long duration aerobic exercise and aerobic exercise combined with high repetition resistance training (Mulvihill and Quigley, 2003).

If the goal is to use exercise as a strategy for obesity reduction, exercise programmes require prescribed energy expenditure of 3000–3500 kcal per week. This would require approximately 45–60 minutes of exercise, for example, purposeful walking performed at a moderate intensity (70% HRmax) on most days of the week (Mulvihill and Quigley, 2003).

FREQUENCY

The frequency remains at 3 to 5 exercise sessions per week, integrating activity into everyday life.

INTENSITY

The intensity for weight management is between 50 and 75% HRmax.

TYPE

Combined cardiovascular (CV) and RE should be included with the aim to increase lean tissue (muscle), as this is more metabolically active.

For overweight patients, avoid high-impact exercises in order to prevent excess stress on joints. Alternatively, non-weightbearing activities could be prescribed, e.g. swimming/water-based activities/cycling. Some obese patients may be embarrassed to do these and some exercise bikes will have a weight restriction. Special consideration should also be given to the individual's ability. (See pp. 117–18 on water-based activities.)

Always ensure alternative exercises are given to accommodate those in the class who are physically unable to carry out certain exercises. In addition, adipose tissue may restrict positions for stretching or the ability to partake in floor-based exercises. Obese patients may have issues with low self-esteem and poor body image. Therefore, the exercise leader should be aware of this and take it into account when prescribing activity to encourage adherence. When monitoring an obese patient it may be difficult to palpate a pulse at the wrist or neck areas, and RPE scales may be the mode of monitoring.

TIME

Increase duration and frequency according to the participant's capacity and aim to increase total energy expenditure.

Diabetes

FITT principles apply as for the post-MI group. Special attention is required for participants who are on insulin or oral hypoglycaemic agents (OHA). Awareness by the exercise leader and participant of the potential for both hypoglycaemia and hyperglycaemia within an exercise situation is essential. Any planned new physical activity should be discussed with the diabetic CR participant and the diabetes care team (Diabetes UK, 2003). After a cardiac event, metabolic stress may induce latent diabetes or can worsen the control of pre-existing diabetes. Therefore, it is essential that diabetes is well controlled prior to the individual commencing exercise. If a participant is newly diagnosed with either type I or type II diabetes, it is advisable that they do not exercise alone until they are able to monitor their response to exercise.

Autonomic and peripheral neuropathies are common in diabetic patients. These neuropathies affect sympathetic and parasympathetic activity, and therefore HR and BP response to exercise may be altered. Sudden changes in position need to be avoided, i.e. lying to standing, in order to avoid orthostatic/postural hypotension.

With peripheral neuropathies, loss of sensation may make pulse palpation difficult, so that RPE scale may be the most appropriate method of monitoring. Gripping of equipment may be problematic due to this poor sensation, and alternatives need to be offered, for example, dumbbells with hand straps. Diabetic patients with peripheral neuropathies may not feel the pain from blisters, so advice should be given to patients on well-fitting training shoes. Feet should be examined regularly, and any friction or nail problems treated immediately or referred to a podiatrist.

Another side effect of diabetes is macro/micro vascular disease. As a result of this, diabetic patients may be more prone to silent ischaemia and peripheral vascular disease. Silent ischaemia may only be detected on their ETT result. Diabetic patients should be closely monitored by the exercise team to assess for increasing breathlessness, which may indicate worsening of their condition in the absence of angina symptoms.

HYPOGLYCAEMIA

Insulin may need to be adjusted on exercise days to avoid hypoglycaemia during or after exercise. Participants should ensure that their exercise partner or exercise leader knows when they are taking their insulin/OHA and what to do in the event of a hypoglycaemic reaction. Insulin regimens can be complicated and must be individualised.

In order to check for signs and symptoms of hypoglycaemia, diabetics on insulin or on OHA should monitor their blood glucose levels before, during and for the first hour or more after exercise. This again should be following advice from the diabetic care team. Delayed hypoglycaemia can occur up to 36 hours after intense activity. This may be avoided by adjusting carbohydrate intake at meal and snack times (Diabetes UK, 2003). Close monitoring is essential, as exercise will alter blood glucose levels. During exercise, the activation of muscle contraction facilitates the uptake of glucose, much like insulin, by making the muscle cells more permeable or allowing glucose to pass into the cells more easily (Ivy, 1987).

For those diabetic participants who inject insulin, the injection site should be standardised and should avoid an exercising limb, since injecting into an exercising muscle may cause the insulin to be absorbed faster than usual. The abdomen area is ideal and least likely to affect performance.

Exercise should be avoided when insulin is at its peak effect. After exercise, the body essentially enters a fasted state, where glycogen stores in muscle and liver are low and hepatic glucose production is accelerated. This is why all diabetic patients on insulin or OHA should have rapidly absorbable glucose drinks and complex carbohydrates readily available, as blood glucose levels can fall during exercise. It is useful to have a selection of these foods and drinks available at all classes.

HYPERGLYCAEMIA

Hyperglycaemia is defined as an abnormally high level of glucose in the blood. If a participant has a blood glucose level >300 mg/L than normal, physical activity should not be undertaken until glucose levels have stabilised. Diabetic specialists should advise participants on how to manage their blood sugar levels and how to test for ketones, which are a byproduct of incomplete metabolism (Diabetes UK, 2003).

Participants need to consult their diabetic care team for advice on adjusting their insulin and carbohydrate intake. As, potentially, exercise intensity continues to progress, ongoing advice should be sought from and provided by the diabetic care team. (See more on diabetes in Chapter 6.)

Peripheral vascular disease (PVD)

FREQUENCY

Exercise should be set at a frequency tolerated by the individual, aiming for three to five times per week, and integrating activity into everyday life.

INTENSITY

This should be dependent on how well exercise is tolerated by the individual. It is more likely that the symptoms of intermittent claudication will limit mobility, rather than the symptoms of coronary heart disease. The exercise should be performed to a level where the PVD patient is 'nudging' the exercise level to the onset of leg pain. With sustained exercise, there is an increase in blood flow to the ischaemic region through capillarisation of the muscles, which will boost exercise tolerance and improve symptoms (ACSM, 2001). Exercise prescribers should use their motivational skills to encourage PVD patients, as they may be anxious about continuing exercise in the onset of PVD pain. PVD scales (ACSM, 2001) can be used to monitor patients while exercising.

TYPE

Walking and lower limb exercise have traditionally been considered the best methods of improving circulation to the lower limbs, but may not be tolerated well by PVD patients. Alternative modes of exercise using non- and partial weightbearing activities, e.g. cycling and rowing, which rarely cause discomfort, can be used to attain the CV exercise dose and possibly to enhance compliance.

TIME

Daily exercise is recommended. Start with short periods and gradually increase duration, as tolerated by PVD individual.

Osteoarthritis/rheumatoid arthritis

FREQUENCY

Exercise in three to five sessions per week are recommended. Patients with rheumatoid arthritis (RA) should be advised not to exercise during periods of exacerbations/flare-ups.

INTENSITY

The intensity should be between 60 and 75% HRmax.

TYPE

This will depend on individuals and their symptoms. Low-impact activities are generally recommended in order to avoid stress on the lower limb joints. Comparable workload intensity to high-impact exercise can be achieved by adding dynamic upper limb exercises to low-impact exercises. Water-based activity may be suitable for arthritis.

Advice should be given regarding good shock-absorbing foot wear, and, if necessary, it may be more appropriate to prescribe non- or partial weight-bearing activities. In addition, patients should be encouraged to develop flexibility and to strengthen muscles around vulnerable joints to encourage joint stability.

TIME

The overload period should last for 20 to 30 minutes.

Osteoporosis

FREQUENCY

Structured exercise for three to five sessions per week. In addition, some form of weight-bearing activity should be advised on a daily basis, along with an active living approach.

INTENSITY

The intensity should be between 50 and 75% HRmax.

TYPE

Weight-bearing exercises are recommended, i.e. stair climbing, brisk walking, stepping. Falls in this group are more likely to result in a fracture, therefore, exercises that encourage strength, balance and coordination should be encouraged. Strengthening should target individual vulnerable sites and postural muscles, such as hip flexors and extensors and back extensors. Exercise leaders should include exercises that will help to develop motor skills and coordination. Care should be taken to avoid making the exercises complicated until motor skills have improved.

TIME

The overload period should last between 20 and 30 minutes.

SUMMARY

This chapter has addressed the components and prescription for exercise and activity for CR across all four phases. Within a cardiac rehabilitation class there will be a wide range of participants, all with varied ability, psychological outlook and preconceptions. The challenge facing the exercise leader and prescriber is complex: to identify co-pathologies and adapt the exercise programme to allow patients to participate safely, yet effectively.

REFERENCES

American Association of Cardiovascular and Pulmonary Rehabilitation (AACVPR) (1999) *Guidelines for Cardiac Rehabilitation and Secondary Prevention Programs*, 3rd edn, Human Kinetics, Champaign, IL.

American College of Sports Medicine (ACSM) (1995) *Guidelines for Exercise Testing and Prescription*, 5th edn, Williams and Wilkins, London.

American College of Sports Medicine (ACSM) (1998) The recommended quantity and quality of exercise for developing and maintaining cardiorespiratory and muscular fitness, and flexibility in healthy adults. *Medicine Science in Sports and Exercise*, **30**, 975–91.

American College of Sports Medicine (ACSM) (2001) *Resource Manual for Guidelines for Exercise Testing and Prescription*, 4th edn, Williams and Wilkins, London.

American Council on Exercise (ACE) (1998) *Exercise for Older Adults*, Human Kinetics, Champaign, IL.

American Heart Association (AHA) (1995) Exercise standards: A statement for health care professionals. *Circulation*, **91**, 580–615.

Anderson, B. (2000) *Stretching: 20th Anniversary*, Shelter Publications, Bolinas, CA.

Anderson, O. (2000). Peak performance – Special Issue. *Sports Injury*, **136**, Peak Performance Publishing, London.

Association of Chartered Physiotherapists in Cardiac Rehabilitation (ACPICR) (1999) *The Chartered Society of Physiotherapy. Standards for the exercise component of Phase III Cardiac Rehabilitation*, The Chartered Society of Physiotherapy, London.

Association of Chartered Physiotherapists in Cardiac Rehabilitation (ACPICR) (2003) *Exercise Physiology and its Application to Exercise Prescription in Cardiac Rehabilitation* – course manual.

Bjarnason-Wehrens, B., Mayer-Berger, W., Meister, E.R., Baum, K., Hambrecht, R., Gielen, S. (2004) Recommendations for resistance exercise in cardiac rehabilitation. Recommendations of the German Federation for Cardiovascular Prevention and Rehabilitation. *European Journal of Cardiovascular Prevention and Rehabilitation*, **11**(4), 352–61.

Blair, S.N., Church, T.S. (2004) The fitness, obesity, and health equation: Is physical activity the common denominator? *Journal of the American Medical Association*, **292**(10), 1232–40.

Boone, W.T., Thompson D.L. (1983) Reproducibility of tethered swimming in exercise rehabilitation research. *American Corrective Therapy*, **37**, 23–7.

Borg, G. (1982) Psychophysical bases of perceived exertion. *Medicine and Science in Sports and Exercise*, **14**, 3337–81.

Borg, G.A.V. (1998) *Borg's Perceived Exertion and Pain Scales*, Human Kinetics, Leeds, Champaign, IL.

British Association for Cardiac Rehabilitation (BACR) (1995) *BACR Guidelines for Cardiac Rehabilitation*, Blackwell Science, Oxford.

British Association for Cardiac Rehabilitation (BACR) (2000) *Cardiac Rehabilitation: An Educational Resource*. Colourways Ltd, London.

British Heart Foundation (BHF) (2001) *Coronary Angioplasty and Coronary Bypass Surgery*, British Heart Foundation, London.

British Heart Foundation (BHF) (2002) *Heart Attack and Rehabilitation*, British Heart Foundation, London.

British Heart Foundation Statistics (BHFS) (2004) http://www.heartstats.org [accessed 19 Nov 2004].

Buckley, J., Holmes, J., Mapp, G. (1999) *Exercise on Prescription: Cardiovascular Activity for Health*, Butterworth Heinemann, Oxford.

Daub, W., Knapik, G., Black, W. (1996) Strength training early after myocardial infarction. *Journal of Cardiopulmonary Rehabilitation*, **16**(2), 108–10.

Diabetes, U.K. (2003) *Physical Activity and Diabetes*, British Diabetic Association, London.

Dimsdale, J.E., Hartley, H., Guiney, T., Ruskin, J.N., Greenblat, D. (1984) Post Exercise Peril: Plasma, catecholamines and exercise. *Journal of the American Medical Association*, **251**, 630–2.

Fardy, P.S., Franklin, B.A., Porcari, J.P., Verrill, D.E. (1998) *Training Techniques in Cardiac Rehabilitation*, Human Kinetics, Leeds.

Fletcher, G.F., Cantwell, J.D., Watt, E.W. (1984) Oxygen consumption and hemodynamic response of exercise used in training of patients with recent myocardial infarction. *Circulation*, **60**, 140–4.

Franklin, B.A. (1993) Easy does it for health. *Fitness Management*, **9**, 41–3.

Health Education Board for Scotland (1997) http://www.hebs.scot.nhs.uk. [accessed 23 Nov 2004]

Ivy, J.L. (1987) The insulin like effect of muscle contraction. *Exercise Sports Science Review*, **15**, 29–51.

Jolliffe, J.A., Rees, K., Taylor, R.S., Thompson, D., Oldridge, N., Ebrahim, S. (2004) Exercise-based rehabilitation for coronary heart disease. *Cochrane Database for Systematic Reviews*.1. [online] available from http://www.cochrane.org [accessed 14 Feb 2004].

Karvonen, M.J., Kentala, F., Mustala, O. (1957) The effects of training on heart rate: A longitudinal study. *Annales Medicinae Experimentalis et Biologiae Fenniae*, **35**, 307–15.

Koszota, L.E. (1989) From sweats to swimsuits: Is water exercise the wave of the future? *Physician and Sports Medicine*, **17**(4), 203–6.

Leon, A.S. (1997) *Physical Activity and Cardiovascular Health: A National Consensus*, Human Kinetics, Leeds.

Lewin, B., Robertson, I.H., Cay, E.L., Irving, J.B., Campbell, M. (1992) Effects of self-help post myocardial-infarction rehabilitation on psychological adjustment and use of health services. *Lancet*, **339**, 1036–40.

Lindsay, G.M., Gaw, A. (1997) *Coronary Heart Disease Prevention: A Handbook for the Health Care Team*, Churchill Livingstone, Edinburgh.

McArdle, W.D., Katch, F.I., Katch, V.L. (1991) *Exercise Physiology: Energy, nutrition and human performance*, 3rd edn, Lea and Febiger, Philadelphia, PA.

Meyer, K. (2001) Exercise training in heart failure: Recommendations based on current research. *Medicine Science in Sport and Exercise*, **33**(4), 525–31.

Mulvihill, C., Quigley, R. (2003) *The Management of Obesity and Overweight: An analysis of reviews of diet, physical activity and behavioural approaches.* Evidence briefing, 1st edn, Health Development Agency.

Pate, R.R., Pratt, M., Blair, S.N., Haskell, W.L., Macera, C.A., Bouchard, C., *et al.* (1995) Physical activity and public health: A recommendation from the Centers for Disease Control and Prevention and the American College of Sports Medicine. *Journal of the American Medical Association*, **273**, 402–7.

Pollock, M.L., Gaesser, G., Butcher, J., Despres, J., Dishman, R., Franklin, B., *et al.* (1998) ACSM position stand: The recommended quantity and quality of exercise for developing and maintaining cardiorespiratory and muscular fitness and flexibility in healthy adults. *Medicine Science in Sport and Exercise*, **30**(6), 975–91.

Pollock, M.L., Franklin, B., Balady, G., Chaitman, B., Fleg, J., Fletcher, B., *et al.* (2000) Resistance exercise in individuals with and without cardiovascular disease: An advisory from the Committee on Exercise, Rehabilitation, and Prevention, Council on Clinical Cardiology, American Heart Association. *Circulation*, **101**(7), 828–33.

Schwade, J., Blomqvist, C.G., Shapiro, W. (1977) A comparison of the leg response to arm and leg work in patients with ischaemic heart disease. *American Heart Journal*, **94**, 203–8.

Scottish Intercollegiate Guidelines Network (SIGN) (2002) *Cardiac Rehabilitation*, no. 57. Edinburgh.

Shvartz, E., Reibold, R.C. (1990) Aerobic fitness norms for males and females aged 6 to 75 years: A review. *Aviation Space Environment Medicine*, **61**, 3–11.

Squires, R.W. (1998) *Exercise Prescription for the High Risk Cardiac Patient*, Human Kinetics, Leeds.

Stickler, T., Malone, T., Garrett, W.E. (1990) The effects of passive warming on muscle injury. *American Journal of Sports Medicine*, **18**(2), 141–5.

Thow, M.K., Armstrong, G., Rafferty, D. (2003) A survey to investigate the non-cardiac conditions and the physiotherapy interventions by physiotherapists in phase III cardiac rehabilitation exercise programs. *Physiotherapy*, **89**(4), 233–7.

Yusuf, S., Cairns, J.A., Camm, J., Falkn, E.L., Gersh, B.J. (2003) *Evidence Based Cardiology*, 2nd edn, BMJ Books, London.

Chapter 5

Class Design and Use of Music in Cardiac Rehabilitation

Linda Harley and Gillian Armstrong

Chapter outline

This chapter focuses on the practical aspects of exercise delivery for phases III and IV group-based exercise classes. Different methods and styles of arranging the group within a space are given to provide interest and variety for the class. In addition, integrating information from previous sections, this chapter explores practical methods for individualising and ideas for progressing exercise prescription. Designing an exercise class requires a good working knowledge of the various physiological responses to exercise and monitoring skills discussed in previous chapters. The components of warm-up (with pulse-raiser, mobility exercises and preparatory stretch), followed by a conditioning component and finally a cool-down incorporating pulse-lowering and developmental stretches are described in order. The use of musculoskeletal endurance exercises as a form of active recovery is discussed. The chapter concludes with advice on the use of music during exercise.

WARM-UP

The warm-up is the preparatory phase of the exercise session. A well-planned and properly executed warm-up improves exercise performance and maximises both the safety and effectiveness of the exercise session. Warm-ups should be at least 15 minutes' duration for cardiac rehabilitation (SIGN, 2002; ACPICR, 2003). This extended time prepares the cardiovascular system for the activity that follows. With this slow, gradual progression of effort, coronary circulation is enhanced (through vasodilation of the coronary arteries), thus

Exercise Leadership in Cardiac Rehabilitation. An Evidence-Based Approach. Edited by Morag Thow.
Copyright 2006 by John Wiley & Sons Ltd. ISBN 0-470-01971-9

reducing the risk of provoking ischaemia and/or arrhythmias. Certain patient groups benefit from an even longer warm-up of up to 20 minutes (e.g. heart transplant recipients, and people with angina).

TYPES OF EXERCISE USED IN A WARM-UP

- Pulse-raising
- Mobilising and preparatory stretching
- Skill rehearsal.

Pulse-raising exercises

Pulse-raising exercises should gradually increase heart rate and blood flow to the active muscles. Pulse-raising exercises involve rhythmic moves, initially of the lower limbs (e.g. marching on the spot, walking forwards and backward, sidestepping, rear step-backs, etc.). These exercises work the large muscle groups aerobically and are performed at a low intensity (i.e. below training heart rate at an RPE ≤ 11 on the original 6–20 scale or ≤ 3 on the modified 0–10 scale). Pulse-raising exercises should be arranged so that there is good transition from one move to the next, so that the exercises flow into one another smoothly. All the moves in the warm-up should be simple to follow and involve minimal skill. Since arm work creates a greater increase in heart rate than leg work, during the warm-up, short lever unilateral movements of the upper limbs are preferred (e.g. shoulder abduction with elbows flexed).

Mobilising exercises

Range of movement exercises such as shoulder lifts and rolls, scapular retractions, trunk side bends, ankle plantar/dorsiflexion, etc. should promote release of synovial fluid into the joint capsule. This will ensure the joints are well lubricated and cushioned. The increased blood flow raises the temperature within the tendons, muscles and ligaments surrounding each joint, improving their viscoelastic properties and allowing fuller range of movement. Preparatory stretches (PS) can be used to assist mobilisation. These should focus on the muscle groups, which are prone to adaptive shortening, either as a result of the ageing process, or as a result of cardiac surgery. With PS the muscle is lengthened to a point where mild tension is experienced and then held still for approximately 10 seconds. While stretches are being performed, it is essential to keep the rest of the body moving to avoid a drop in heart rate or venous pooling. There continues to be some debate on the benefits of PS in the athletic population (Thacker, *et al.*, 2004) for the CR group it seems prudent to continue with PS.

Skill rehearsal

During the warm-up to assist in motor learning the aerobic and stretching exercise performed should include some of the activities that will be used in the main overload period. This gives the participants a chance to rehearse the moves and to start learning motor skills by repeating them.

Key points on warm-up for exercise leader

- Start with small mobility and pulse-raising exercises and **gradually** build up the range of motion and intensity of the movements.
- Keep all steps low impact and minimal skill.
- Ensure the body is completely warm before stretching.
- Combine preparatory stretches with pulse-raising exercises to prevent venous pooling and the heart rate dropping.
- Use moves in the warm-up that will be repeated in the overload and cool-down to allow rehearsal and motor learning.

CARDIOVASCULAR OVERLOAD COMPONENT

Definition

To elicit a beneficial physiological effect, the cardiovascular (CV) system must be stressed above a normal level of exertion. This is sometimes referred to as the training threshold or zone. The training threshold is influenced by many factors (including a person's current aerobic capacity and training status). In sedentary and deconditioned individuals, it may be as low as 55% HRmax (ACSM, 1998) (see more in Chapter 4).

KEY POINTS

The conditioning component should:

- principally be CV work, involving rhythmic movement of the main large muscle groups of the upper and lower body;
- last approximately 20–30 minutes;
- initially adopt an interval approach;
- vary in the length of CV work and active recovery intervals until gradually progressing to continuous CV exercise;
- use progression of intensity as appropriate;
- consider the needs of the novice exerciser with low self-efficacy.

Rationale for interval training

The premise of interval training is that an individual can produce a greater amount of work in a training session if the training bouts are spaced between periods of lower intensity work. Usually these active recovery (AR) periods are between 30 seconds and one minute in duration (see Chapter 4).

KEY POINTS ON ACTIVE RECOVERY EXERCISES

- lower intensity cardiovascular activity, e.g. walking;
- musculoskeletal endurance (MSE) work, e.g. exercises to improve local endurance of muscles NOT used in the cardiovascular stations.

PROGRESSION FROM INTERVAL TO CONTINUOUS CV WORK

In this context continuous can mean that the AR is removed, or that the subject participates in one mode, e.g. rowing or cycling for the entire overload section. The goal is to progress participants from interval to continuous training as their fitness improves. The duration of the active recovery sections must be either reduced or maintained. Aerobic activity can be altered either through increased durations of CV work or through an increase in intensity. This will depend on an individual's risk stratification and rehabilitation goals.

WHY CIRCUITS?

Circuits (circuits in this context do not refer to circuit training) have become the most popular mode of delivery in cardiac rehabilitation because they can be designed without a large amount of equipment. A further advantage is that circuits offer variety, and each station can be adapted to allow for individual ability, thus allowing progression both within and between stations. In addition, they provide motor skills development and include more functional-type exercise. Furthermore, circuits are an opportunity for social interaction amongst participants and, because the exercise leader is not required to exercise, he or she is free to move around participants and to provide individual coaching and correction. Finally, depending on the type of circuits created, they can be used as a model for home-based exercise. Home-based exercise circuits can be delivered as a video or using copies of the stations on the *Physiotools* package (2005) with a created handout of individual exercises.

FACTORS TO CONSIDER IN CIRCUIT DESIGN

Careful planning and preparation, knowing in advance the limitations on room size, equipment available, number of participants, etc. will all help make the circuit design work in practice. In general the circuit must follow in a logical sequence with an easy-to-follow plan. This becomes more important especially with larger groups and with participants of different levels of exercise ability, for example, from very deconditioned to above average fitness.

Most circuits include 8 to 12 exercise stations. Your circuit needs to have a sufficient number of stations to accommodate all the participants, along with sufficient trained staff to supervise those exercising. Current Association of Chartered Physiotherapists in Cardiac Rehabilitation (ACPICR, 2003) guidelines recommend a staff-to-patient ratio of 1 : 5. You need to pre-plan how staff will monitor stations effectively, e.g. take responsibility for three or four stations, or responsibility for four or five people moving round the entire circuit. If you are planning to use exercise equipment you will have to make sure there is enough available to prevent queuing as participants wait for equipment to become available. Above all you need to ensure that the circuit consists of adequate aerobic-type exercises (see Table 5.1) and includes different ways of adjusting the exercise intensity (see Table 5.2) without introducing high-impact moves.

Table 5.1. Examples of aerobic exercise

Leg Pattern	Arm Pattern
Knee lifts	Elbow bends
Toe taps behind	Double punch forwards
Toe taps to side	Side arm raises
Knee bends	Butterfly (pectoral)
Back heel lifts	Criss-cross to front
Three steps forwards and back	Arm raise above head
Side lunges	Hand push-downs
Heel digs to front	Reach pull back
March	Forward elbow circles
Two steps to side and back	Low swing behind back
Step kicks	Diagonal arm reaches
Toe taps to front	Forward arm swing

Table 5.2. Methods of altering intensity of an aerobic exercise

Range of movement (e.g. step height, step length)
Speed of movement
Length of levers (upper limb)
Unilateral / bilateral movement
Plane of movement (above/below chest height)
Change load (hold light hand dumbbells)
Change exercise duration

CHOICE AND ARRANGEMENT OF STATIONS

In order to maximise the desirable physiological effect, the majority of the exercises should be aerobic in nature. Aerobic exercises involve rhythmic movement of large muscle groups involving the whole body. Variations in the starting position of an upper body exercise can have a significant effect on rate pressure product (RPP). For example, elbow flexion and extension performed with the arms by the side are easier than when the arms are held at shoulder level, which is easier than when the arms are held high above the head.

When selecting individual exercises, it is essential to ensure there is a balance of exercise on different muscle groups, and that consecutive exercises do not result in overusing any one muscle group (e.g. step-ups followed by cycling will result in excessive quadriceps work).

Active recovery stations, by their very nature, need to be evenly spaced amongst the aerobic stations and not next to one another. AR exercise involves a muscle to exert sub-maximal forces against a resistance over an extended period of time and differs from strength. Musculoskeletal endurance (MSE) is best developed by using lighter weights and with a greater number of repetitions (Pollock, *et al.*, 1998). As a rule for muscular endurance, select resistances that allow more than 16 repetitions to be performed without inducing fatigue (i.e. RPE less than 15). AR are generally used to increase endurance of specific muscle groups, e.g. quadriceps, and are of a lower intensity, i.e. 60% HRmax. If muscular endurance exercises are chosen, then they should target muscles not used extensively in the CV component (see Table 5.3 for some examples).

A useful website resource for theraband (http://www.thera-bandacademy.com) provides a database of exercises using elastic bands and allows you to create a printed handout.

Table 5.3. Examples of muscular endurance exercises

Muscle/group	Exercise
Gastrocnemius	Standing single calf raises
Gluteals	Standing single hip extension
Upper trapezius and deltoid	Upright row holding weighted pole
Lateral dorsi and rhomboids	Seated row with elastic band
Triceps	Standing press backs or seated dips
Gluteal medius and minimus	Standing hip abduction
Biceps	Bicep curls holding dumbbells
Lateral rotator cuff	Seated shoulder rotations with elastic band
Quadriceps, hamstrings and gluteal maximus	Wallslides
Pectorals and triceps	Chest press (band around back under arms)

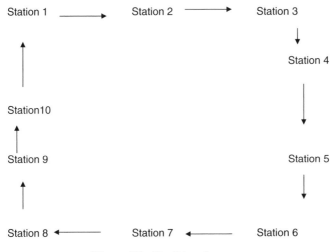

Figure 5.1. Traditional square.

ROOM ARRANGEMENT

In its basic format, a circuit is usually arranged around the perimeter of the room (see Figure 5.1).

Alternative layouts, which may better suit the dimensions of the exercise room, are shown in Figures 5.2 to 5.6. Using different room arrangements provides variety, while still using the same stations.

Often circuit classes are held in physiotherapy departments, where other equipment is stored. Figure 5.4a and 5.4b circuit arrangement gets round the problem of participants finding themselves crammed into the corners. In Figure 5.4b only four stations are displayed at any one time then the circuit cards are changed to display four different stations. This is helpful when there are several beginners in the class as it keeps it simple for both the participants and the instructor. Participants follow the circuit in order of the numbers.

In circuit 5.5 the whole group is split into two smaller groups. One group goes round the perimeter stations in a clockwise direction, while the other group goes round the perimeter stations in an anticlockwise direction. This means that participants exercise with a different person at each station, rather than going round the whole circuit with the same person. This can be a useful way of getting the group to mix and it can promote better self-pacing and less competiveness, since the exercise partner is constantly changing.

Circuit 5.6 works best in a long hall, when class sizes are bigger and exercises are all aerobic in nature. The group is split into four or more smaller groups which remain in a line. Each group starts with a different exercise, moving from group A to E. Participants look along to the next line on their right for the next exercise. The line at the far end (line E) will not be able to

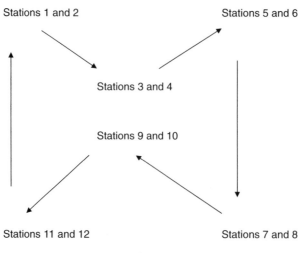

Figure 5.2. Bow tie circuit.

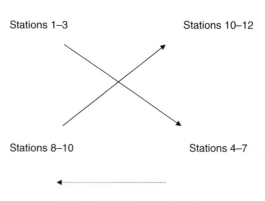

Figure 5.3. Corners circuit.

see the start line so the exercise leader has to demonstrate. After all five exercises have been completed the exercise leader gets the group to perform an active recovery walk and then changes the line exercise for the second circuit. This circuit relies on at least one participant in each group acting as a line leader.

STATION DURATION

Aerobic stations can vary between 30 seconds and three minutes, with the duration dictated by participants' functional capacity. Least fit participants will

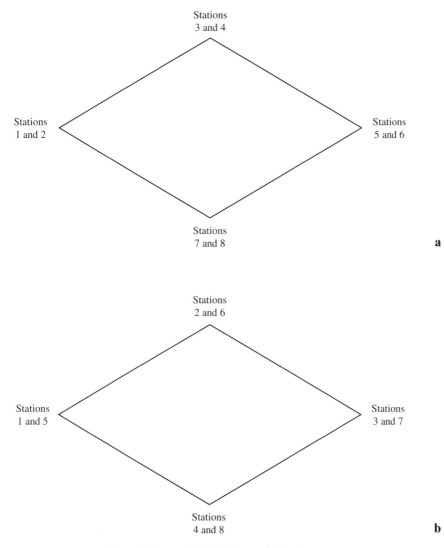

Figure 5.4a. and 5.4b. Diamond circuits.

need a much more defined interval approach than will fitter participants (see rationale for interval training p. 135).

Active recovery stations should last for no more than one minute. The time between consecutive stations should be kept to a minimum, and, as a guide, should only last long enough for participants to walk from one station to the next. Different ways of controlling the circuit time and movement are discussed later in this chapter.

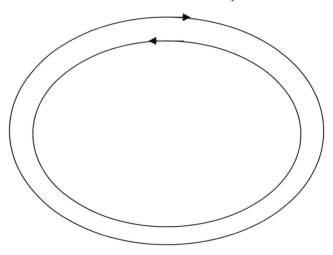

Figure 5.5. Concentric circles circuit.

Group	A	B	C	D	E
	☺	☺	☺	☺	☺
	☺	☺	☺	☺	☺
	☺	☺	☺	☺	☺
	☺	☺	☺	☺	☺

Figure 5.6. Line circuit.

Mat or floor work should never be included in the main circuit. During aerobic exercise training, exercises which involve lying down are contraindicated for several reasons. Lying down creates a sudden increase in the volume of blood returning to the heart (preload). This causes an increase in the left ventricular end diastolic volume, which could cause arrhythmias and angina. Second, there is a risk of orthostatic hypotension when returning to upright posture. In cardiac patients, ACE inhibitors, nitrates and beta blockers may exacerbate this. Finally, participants may have physical difficulty getting up and down and, with a limited time at each station, this can result in participants not adopting the correct starting position or not performing exercises correctly. If exercises on the floor are to be included, they should be used after the cool-down.

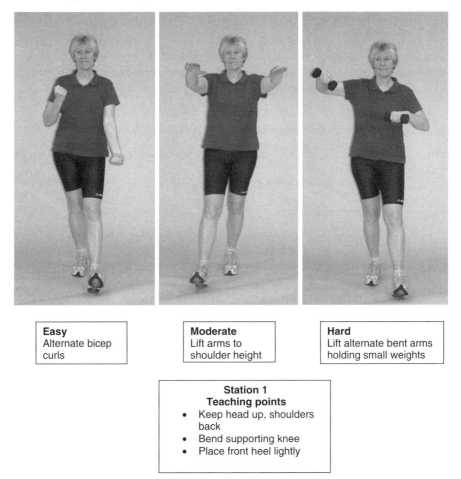

| Easy
Alternate bicep
curls | Moderate
Lift arms to
shoulder height | Hard
Lift alternate bent arms
holding small weights |

Station 1
Teaching points
- Keep head up, shoulders back
- Bend supporting knee
- Place front heel lightly

Figure 5.7. Example of a circuit chart. The heel dig is the basic step, with arm pattern providing increasing intensity.

USE OF CIRCUIT AND RPE TRAINING CARDS

Circuit cards act as a prompt but can never replace proper instruction. They can be colour coded for easy recognition – e.g. to identify different intensities or types of exercise (see Figure 5.7). When used, circuit cards must have the following characteristics:

- clearly visible and identifiable (ideally A2 size);
- numbered;
- include large, clear diagrams;

- with minimal text – only key teaching points;
- laminated.

In addition to circuit cards, there should be an RPE scale of the same size beside the circuit card. The exercise leader and assistants can refer the patients to the appropriate self-monitoring during the class.

CLASS MANAGEMENT: CONTROL OF CLASS MOVEMENT

The control of the circuits also needs to be carefully considered, as it can be done in a number of ways.

Time control

- Exercise leader uses a stopwatch and calls out prescribed times to stop, start and move on to the next exercise.
- Exercise leader uses stop watch, blows a whistle when it is time to change.
- Exercise leader uses pre-recorded tapes, where the work time at each station and changeover times are controlled by recording the playing time and breaks in the music.

Repetition control

This method uses one of the stations to dictate time. For example, a pre-set number of shuttle walks completed by participants at one station is the cue for the whole group to move on to the next station. Alternatively, the exercise leader prescribes individuals with a set number of repetitions to complete before moving on to the next station, e.g. 8, 12, 16 or 20 of each exercise. This method is not often adopted in CR programmes, as it may result either in participants rushing through the exercises (thus at an inappropriate intensity) or all finishing their conditioning component at different times. However, it can be employed effectively in an unsupervised home programme.

EXAMPLES OF PHASE III CIRCUIT FORMAT AND THEIR PROGRESSIONS

Figure 5.8 and Table 5.4 show a format that would be ideal in a gym situation, where there is a small number of participants and a selection of different types of CV equipment.

Here the aerobic exercise stations alternate with a lower intensity aerobic exercise (walking). The lower intensity walking between stations acts as an active recovery. The timings used in this circuit work only when using cardiovascular machines, where it is preferable to have a longer duration. The total time for one circuit is 12 minutes. Participants need to go round the circuit twice in order to achieve the standard training duration.

Table 5.4. Example of phase III circuit and progression with CV equipment

Different stages	CV time	AR time
Stage 1: Perform 1 minute at each station, then 1 minute of walking around gym, before moving on to next station.	6 mins	6 mins
Stage 2: Perform $1^1/_2$ minutes at each station, then $^1/_2$ minute of walking around gym, before moving on to next station.	9 mins	3 mins
Stage 3: Perform 2 minutes at each station before moving on to next station.	12 mins	0

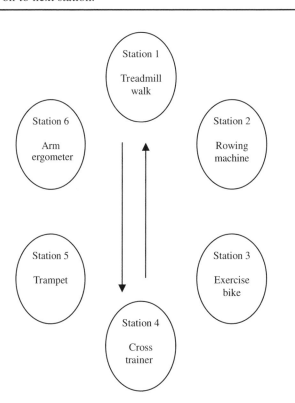

Figure 5.8. Circuit format with CV equipment.

ADVANTAGES OF FIGURE 5.8

- It is easily adopted in a fitness studio environment.
- There are fewer stations, making the circuit straightforward to follow. Circuit progresses through duration first.
- The small number of stations allows the exercise leader to move around and observe the group more easily (important when using CV machines, where there is a risk of injury/misuse).
- Fewer stations make it is easier for the exercise leader to manage and for beginners to learn the circuit.
- The use of CV equipment allows the exercise leader to alter the workload more exactly (better individualisation). Less time urgency, so that participants can focus more on their exercise technique, sensation of effort, etc.
- Longer time intervals at each station mean that the exercise leader has more opportunity to talk to participants and offer teaching points without interruption.
- Less competitive – participants are not as rushed to get started because they know they have a reasonable length of time in which to settle into the exercise.

DISADVANTAGE OF FIGURE 5.8

- With this circuit arrangement, unless there is more than one item of gym equipment per station, the number of participants is limited to six.
- Due to the small number of stations, it may become repetitive or boring for participants.
- Exercise leader may become complacent and simply operate as a timekeeper.
- There is no MSE work within the circuit.
- Exercise leader has to provide separate individual induction for all equipment.
- New participants may need a lot of help with programming the equipment and, for example, altering the seat position of a bicycle.
- The order of the stations may be fixed because the equipment cannot be moved around the room.
- The exercise durations will not work well for participants with a very low functional capacity or a mobility problem.

Figure 5.9 and Table 5.5 show aerobic stations with MSE exercises as an active recovery. The even numbered stations are aerobic, while the odd numbered stations are active recovery. Progression is achieved by increasing CV time at the expense of the AR time. It is advisable to change the aerobic stations before the start of the third circuit, to prevent boredom. Participants must keep feet moving while performing upper body exercises. The total time for one circuit is six minutes 20 seconds. Participants need to go round the circuit three to four times in order to achieve the standard training duration.

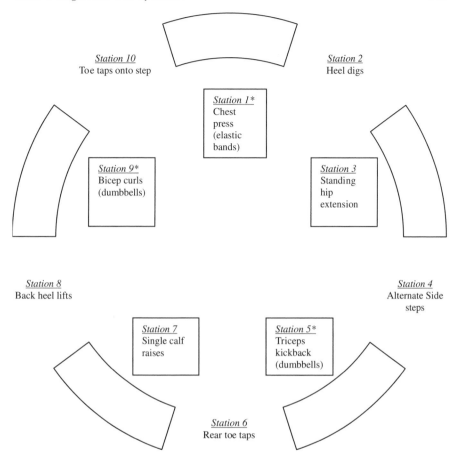

Figure 5.9. Circuit showing aerobic stations with MSE exercises as an active recovery.
  * Keep feet moving entire time.

Table 5.5. Example of phase III circuit and progression with aerobic and AR using MSE stations

Stages	CV time	AR time
Stage 1 Perform 40 seconds of exercise at all stations.	3 mins 10 secs	3 mins 10 secs
Stage 2 Perform 60 seconds of exercise at the even numbered stations and 20 seconds of exercise at the odd numbered stations.	5 mins	1 min 20 secs
Stage 3 Perform 1 minute 20 seconds at the even numbered stations and miss out all the odd numbered stations.	6 mins 20 secs	0

ADVANTAGES OF FIGURE 5.9

- Plenty of variety of exercises can be included.
- Plan can accommodate a greater number of patients, before having to double up at stations.
- It can cater for a wide variety of fitness levels, provided progression options are clearly stated.
- It does not require aerobic exercise equipment.
- The active recovery period incorporates MSE work.
- Circuit can be arranged in different ways according to the dimension of the room.

DISADVANTAGES OF FIGURE 5.9

- Plan requires a large area of floor space.

- More stations = more time-consuming to set up at the start.
- Timings may be confusing, especially for novices.
- There is less opportunity for MSE work as the participants progress. (If the AR time is not reduced as the CV time increases, participants move on at different times, and consequently there could be a bottleneck at some stations.)
- More staff are required, in order to provide adequate supervision at each station.
- Patients are more likely to perform the MSE exercises at the speed of an aerobic exercise (especially when using music), thereby not providing active recovery.

Figure 5.10 and Tables 5.6 and 5.7 show aerobic stations with MSE exercises as an active recovery. There are 12 stations, and at each station there is a choice of an aerobic or an active recovery exercise. The circuit cards are colour coded so that they are easily identifiable (e.g. green = aerobic, red = active recovery). Beginners are told to alternate between green and red exercises. The exercise duration at each station is fixed at 45 seconds, with 10 seconds allowed for changeover to next station. If the circuit is performed once then the training period is approximately 10 minutes. If it is repeated, this would give a training period of approximately 20 minutes. The circuit would need to be repeated three times in order to produce a training period of approx 30 minutes. Alternatively, a 10-minute exercise to music section could be used instead of a third circuit. Progression is then achieved by substituting an AR station with an aerobic station. Total time for one circuit is nine minutes. Participants need to go round the circuit three to four times in order to achieve the standard training duration.

ADVANTAGES OF FIGURE 5.10

- Timings are straightforward – everyone moves at the same time, prevents queuing when there is more of a chance of participants standing waiting.

- Variety of stations prevents boredom and accommodates a wide variety of fitness levels.
- Circuit cards act as prompts and reinforce good technique.

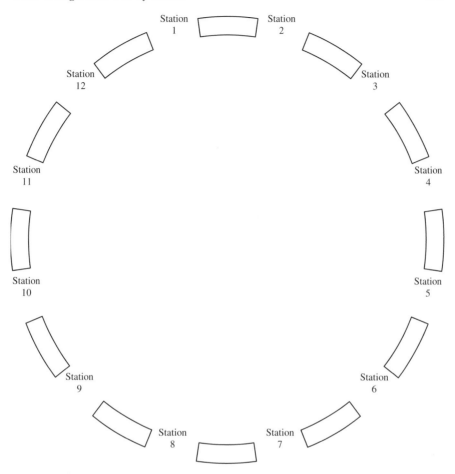

Figure 5.10. Circuit showing aerobic stations with MSE exercises as an active recovery.

DISADVANTAGES OF FIGURE 5.10

- Plan requires considerable group management skills.
- Individual participants have to remember what type of work to do at each station (i.e. aerobic or active recovery work) and not just copy what the person ahead of them is doing.
- If there is more than one person per station, it may be confusing if they are doing different exercises.

Table 5.6. Example of phase III circuit and progression with colour-coded aerobic and AR using MSE stations

Stages	CV time	AR time
Stage 1 Perform 1 (green) aerobic station followed by 1 (red) active recovery station	4.5 mins	4.5 mins
Stage 2 Perform 2 (green) aerobic stations followed by 1 (red) active recovery station	6 mins	3 mins
Stage 3 Perform 5 (green) aerobic stations followed by 1 (red) active recovery station	7.5 mins	1.5 mins
Stage 4 Perform all 12 (green) aerobic stations	9 mins	0

Table 5.7. Aerobic stations and MSE stations: examples of exercises

Station Number	CV option	AR option
1	Side lunges off low step with half arm swing	Half squat (back against wall)
2	Shoulder pulley above head*	Theraband shoulder pull back*
3	Knee lifts + butterfly (pectorals)	Walk around gym
4	Heel digs + forward arm lifts	Bicep curls while slow walking around gym
5	Shuttle walk	Theraband hip extension (looped band secured around bottom rung of wallbars)
6	Elbow circles with step kicks	Theraband shoulder diagonal extension*
7	Tap backs behind with shoulder girdle retractions	Hand on wall, hip abductions 5 one leg (turn round then rpt with opposite leg)
8	Alternate arm diagonals with step touch	Theraband shoulder lateral rotation*
9	Box step – passing small ball around body at waist height	Shoulder abductions holding dumbbells*
10	Hamstring curl with upright row	Standing calf raises and toe raises
11	Low march on spot	Overhead shoulder llift*
12	Shuttle walk	Triceps kickback holding dumbbells*

*Keep feet moving entire time.

Figure 5.11 and Table 5.8 show aerobic stations followed by command led MSE station.

This circuit is a modified concentric circles arrangement. The outer circuit is made up of 10 aerobic stations (1–10). Circuit cards on the wall act as aids for the outer circuit. Class exercise leader walks around perimeter of the room to observe patients. During the aerobic circuit, active recovery is incorporated

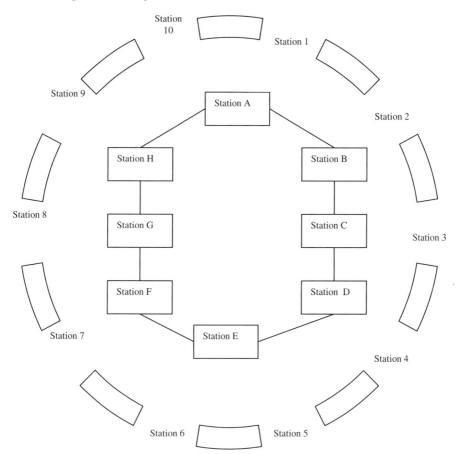

Figure 5.11. Circuit showing aerobic and command MSE.

by reducing the intensity of the aerobic exercise according to the needs of the patient. The outer circuit is completed once, followed by an active recovery walk to allow heart rate to reduce before performing MSE work. The inner circuit is made up of 8 different MSE exercises (A–H) that are command led.

ADVANTAGES OF FIGURE 5.11

- It is fairly simple to teach
- It is very flexible.
- The large variety of aerobic stations keeps participants interested.

- All the patients perform the MSE work at the same time for the same number of reps and are taught by the exercise leader who is able to reinforce all the teaching points.

Table 5.8. Aerobic and command MSE

Cardiovascular stations	Musculoskeletal endurance stations
Station 1 Heel digs with forward arm reach	MSE station A – Standing L hip abduction holding onto chair
Station 2 Rear tap backs with bicep curls	MSE station B – Standing R hip extension
Station 3 March on spot with above-head arm raise every 4th count	MSE station C – Standing calf raises
Station 4 Side tap with short lever arm abduction	MSE station D – Standing L hip extension
Station 5 3 steps forward then heel strike then 3 steps backwards then heel strike	MSE station E – Standing R hip abduction
Station 6 Alternate knee raises (hand to opposite knee)	MSE station F – Seated chest press with elastic band (triceps and pectorals) (continue with heel lifts)
Station 7 Forward toe taps	MSE station G – Seated shoulder lateral rotations with elastic bands (continue with alternate heel lifts)
Station 8 Side steps – 2 to the left then 2 to the right	MSE station H – Seated abdominals (continue with ankle dorsiflexions)
Station 9 Half squat	
Station 10 Back heel lifts	

- For the command-led circuit (no cards needed, easy to offer alternatives, instructor always does the easiest version)

- If using music then the bpm selected can match the type of exercise being performed.

Disadvantages of Figure 5.11

- It needs a large floor space to accommodate all 10 stations and have space for staff to observe participants and correct when needed.
- If circuit cards are stuck on the wall, then patients do the exercises facing the wall!
- In order to keep class management simple, progression of the aerobic workload is achieved by increasing intensity rather than duration, otherwise beginners will finish the circuit before the rest of the class. This may not be a problem if you have a second exercise leader to take them through their MSE work and cool-down.

Figure 5.12 and Tables 5.9 and 5.10 show aerobic circuit with alternative method of controlling exercise time. In this layout, all the stations are aerobic in nature. Circuit cards are pinned on the wall at eye level. Each circuit card shows two options: one to make the intensity lower and the other to make the intensity harder.

Station 9 is the time-controlling station, e.g. 10 step-ups leading with right leg, then go to another step to do 10 step-ups leading with left leg.

Participants at station 9 are given a hooter and perform a preset number of repetitions that has been calculated to take the majority of participants one minute to complete. Once completed, the participant finishing at station 9 sounds the hooter to cue the rest of the class to move on to the next station, before handing over to next person. Total time for one circuit is ten minutes. Participants need to go round the circuit three to four times in order to achieve the standard training duration.

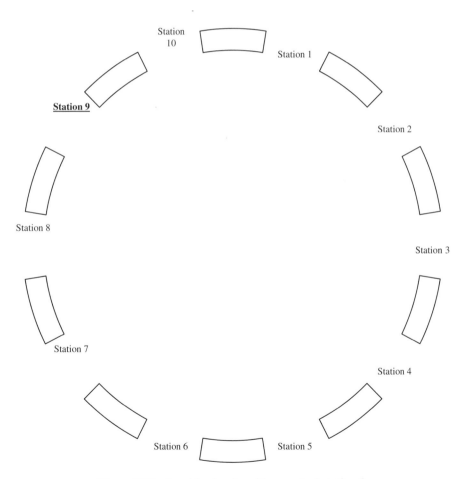

Figure 5.12. Aerobic circuits with a control station **9**.

Table 5.9. Aerobic circuit of 1 minute stations

Stages	CV time	AR time
Stage 1 – Do 2 circuits then 2 minute walk between circuits	20 mins	2 mins
Stage 2 – Do 3 circuits then 2 minute walk between circuits	30 mins	4 mins

Table 5.10. Variety of exercises with options for each station

Station	Exercise	Option 1 (lower)	Option 2 (higher)
1	Knee lift with hand to opposite knee	Hands rest on hips	Hand to opposite shin
2	Step back with tricep kickback	Alternate calf raises instead of step back	Take larger steps
3	Half squat with single arm reach across body	Only do arm reach every 4th count	Hold light dumbbells
4	Hamstring curl with bilateral bicep curls	Toe tap behind	Substitute bicep curls with chest press
5	Heel dig with pec dec keeping elbows high	Elbows lower, hands at eye level	Alternate between 4 pec decs then 4 punches above head
6	Side toe taps with arm swing across body	Hands rest on hips	Pass softball around body
7	March on spot with shoulder retractions	Substitute leg work with alternate heel lifts, keep same arm work	Jog on spot and punch
8	Box step, hands in/out at chest height	Change arm work to bicep curl	Change to arm raises above head
9	10 step-ups (L leg leading) at one end of room (toe taps onto step, easier) instead use higher step then shuttle walk to other step to do another 10 step-ups (R leg leading) – ×2		
10	2 sidesteps with bilateral forward flexion arm lift	Single arm lifts instead	Increase speed of arm work to arm pump

ADVANTAGES OF FIGURE 5.12

- Keeps all participants interested and involved.
- Exercise leader is not tied up with timings and can spend time inducting new participants

DISADVANTAGES OF FIGURE 5.12

- Fitter participants will finish the controlling station sooner, and therefore the exercise time will be less than desired (and vice versa).
- If there are more stations than participants, there will be periods when no one is available to do the timings.
- There is no MSE work in the circuit.
- This may encourage competitiveness between participants.

COOL-DOWN

A cool-down is a period of at least 10 minutes of diminishing intensity exercise and stretching performed immediately after completion of the circuit. The lower intensity exercise gradually returns patients to their pre-exercise state with less risk of hypotension, arrhythmias or angina.

There is a moderate risk of arrhythmia during the period immediately following cessation of exercise because sympathetic activity is still raised. In Van Camp and Peterson's study of 20 cardiac arrests (1989) 30% of cardiac arrests occurred during the cool-down and 10% after the exercise session. Thus, care and monitoring of participants are important during and after the cool-down session.

Older adults have an increased risk of hypotension due to an age-related slowing of baroreceptor responsiveness. There is also an increased risk of venous pooling, as an older adult's HR takes longer to return to pre-exercise state.

Current ACPICR (2003) standards for the phase III exercise component of cardiac rehabilitation stipulate an observation period of at least 15 minutes from the end of the cool-down period, during which relaxation can be taught or education sessions delivered.

Flexibility and stretching

In the cool-down, developmental stretches of the main muscle groups are held for up to 30 seconds (ACSM, 2000). The exercise leader must have sound knowledge of the normal physiological range of movement around the specific joint(s) in order to teach effective stretches. It is also essential to teach supported positions to promote relaxation and allow effective stretching (but not on the floor), for example, quads stretch done while holding or leaning against a wall.

The advice to patients is to stretch until they feel a certain amount of discomfort associated with the stretched position, but no pain. During the stretch normal relaxed breathing should be maintained. As the stretch is held, stress-relaxation occurs, and the force within the muscle decreases. When patients feel less tension because of changes in viscoelasticity they can relax further into the stretch.

Most clinicians believe ballistic stretching increases the risk of injury, because the muscle may reflexly contract if restretched quickly following a short relaxation period. Thus, static stretches are advocated for CR classes.

SPECIAL CONSIDERATIONS IN CARDIAC REHABILITATION POPULATION
FOR STRETCHING

- Adaptive shortening of muscles due to sternotomy wound (especially of pectorals, shoulder lateral rotators and extensors)
- Valsalva manoeuvre, holding breath
- Marfan's syndrome.

Stretching for surgical patients should focus on the muscles that may have adaptive shortening. In addition, during stretching relaxed breathing should be encouraged and the exercise leader should reinforce the avoidance breath holding.

Marfan's syndrome is a inherited condition that affects the connective tissue. The primary purpose of connective tissue is to hold the body together and provide a framework for growth and development. In Marfan's syndrome, the connective tissue is defective and does not act as it should (decreased ligamentous support). Marfan's syndrome affects many organ systems. Some patients with Marfan's syndrome develop aortic valve problems and require replacement valve surgery. Defective connective tissue also results in either joint laxity (hypermobility) or contractures (hypomobility). Care should be taken with this group so as to prevent damage to joint structures.

MUSIC IN CR

Music is commonly used in exercise situations. Music provides some or all of the following:

- creates atmosphere;
- can motivate;
- can be used to dictate time of circuits;
- can be used to choreograph free aerobics.

See Table 5.11 for pros and cons of music.

Table 5.11. Pros and cons of music

Pros	Cons
• motivating • helps create right atmosphere • sets the pace for the exercise • improves mood	• participants may not be able to hear instructions/teaching points • participants try to exercise at the tempo of the music

Phonographic performance limited (PPL) licence

It is important to check the copyright position of recorded music before it is used during cardiac rehabilitation sessions. PPL is the UK record industry royalty collection society. Before you use music in an exercise session, you must obtain a PPL licence. Two rates apply, depending on the number of classes you take. Some companies produce non-PPL licensed music. However, the songs are not performed by the original artists (found at http://www.ppluk.com 2004).

Music tempo

The speed of music is measured in beats per minute (bpm). It is important that you choose music appropriate for the exercise that you want participants to do.

Appropriate tempos for a cardiac rehab exercise class are:

- Warm-up   110–126 bpm
- CV component   126–136 bpm
- Cool-down   118–122 bpm
- MSE   100–110 bpm
- Relaxation   <100 bpm.

Musical structure

The beats in music make up a pattern known as a phrase. Working with the phrasing helps cueing and determines when movements should start, stop and change. Most pre-recorded exercise-to-music tapes and CDs are arranged in phrases with eight beats. For instance, the verse may have four sets of eight beats and the chorus two sets of eight beats.

CHOREOGRAPHY AND FREE AEROBICS

Aerobic overload can be delivered using free aerobics. This method sees the exercise leader perform the exercise with the class following the demonstration and cueing of the exercises. The leader should provide alternatives, giving easy and harder options for each exercise. This style of aerobics within the overload section may not be appropriate early in phase III CR until patients have mastered self-monitoring.

In free aerobics (exercise to music), where the leader is introducing different combinations and moves with music, the leader is required to link and combine exercises with an element of choreography. Free aerobics is often the method used in the warm-up section. Free aerobics (FA) has some disadvantages:

- It is more difficult to control intensity;
- Monitoring patients/participants is more difficult;
- It is harder to provide alternative moves;
- Position and proximity of the participants require close attention.

The advantages of FA include:

- The cost is low;
- There is no need for equipment;
- More motor skill balance and co-ordination are required by the group and leader;
- More independence is required of participants.

The exercise leader performs the skill of structuring foot and arm patterns to the beat and phrase of the music. Usually all steps are choreographed to a 32-count beat.

The most basic method of choreography is to do one foot/arm pattern for eight counts, a second one for eight counts, a third for eight counts and a fourth for eight counts. The first beat of each phrase tends to be the strongest one, and it is this one that should be used to start a new move.

Moves should be taught in counts of 2s, 4s or 8s, e.g. single side-step, double side-step, 4 side-steps, etc. Choosing odd numbers of moves will result in your losing the natural phrasing. See more in Chapter 7 for teaching skills of choreography.

Effect of music on RPE

Thornby, *et al.* (1995) found that COPD patients exercising with music reported a reduced sense of effort (measured as rate of perceived exertion RPE). Music was found to improve mood during aerobic exercise (Seath and Thow 1995). More recently Murrock (2002) found that playing upbeat music during cardiac rehabilitation exercise sessions did not reduce perceived exertion but significantly enhanced mood (measured on a feelings scale).

SUMMARY

This chapter has described the practical aspects of design and delivery of group exercise, using both circuits and free aerobics. It is the choice and preference for the exercise leader as to which method they use. Both methods have strengths and weaknesses. The use of music is also at the discretion of the leader, either as background to dictate circuit time, or to use with the free aerobics section.

REFERENCES

American College of Sports Medicine (ACSM) (1998) Position Stand: The recommended quantity and quality of exercise for developing and maintaining cardiorespiratory and muscular strength and flexibility in healthy adults. *Medicine and Science in Sports and Exercise*, **30**, 975–91.

American College of Sports Medicine (ACSM) (2000) *Guidelines for Exercise Testing and Prescription*, 6th edn, Lippincott, Williams and Wilkins, Baltimore, MD.

Association of the Chartered Physiotherapists Interested in Cardiac Rehabilitation (ACPICR) (2003) *Standards for the Exercise Component of the Phase III Cardiac Rehabilitation*, The Chartered Society of Physiotherapy, London.

Murrock, C.J. (2002) The effect of music on the rate of perceived exertion and general mood among coronary artery bypass graft patients enrolled in cardiac rehabilitation phase 2. *Rehabilitation Nursing*, **27**(6), 227–31.

Physiotools © 2005 Finland.

Pollock, M.L., Gaesser, G.A., Butcher, J.D., Després, J.P., Dishman, R.K., Franklin, B.A., *et al.* (1998) American College of Sports Medicine Position Stand. The recommended quantity and quality of exercise for developing and maintaining cardiorespiratory and muscular fitness, and flexibility in healthy adults. *Medicine and Science in Sport and Exercise*, **30**(6), 975–91.

PPL licence (2004) http://www.ppluk.com [accessed 12 Nov 2004].

Scottish Intercollegiate Guidelines Network (SIGN) (2002) *Cardiac Rehabilitation*, no. 57. Edinburgh.

Seath, L., Thow, M. (1995) The effect of music on the perception of effort and mood during aerobic type exercise. *Physiotherapy*, **81**(10), 592–96.

Thacker, S.B., Gilchrist, J., Stroup, D.F., Kimsey, D. (2004) The impact of stretching on sports injury risk: A systematic review of the literature. *Medicine and Science in Sport and Exercise*, **36**(3), 371–78.

Theraband Academy (http://www.thera-bandacademy.com) [accessed 21 Nov 2004].

Thornby. A., Haas, F., Axen, K.P. (1995) Effect of distractive auditory stimuli on exercise tolerance in patients with COPD. *Chest*, **107**(5), 213–17.

Van Camp, S.P., Peterson, R.A. (1989) Identification of the high-risk cardiac rehabilitation patient. Journal *of Cardiopulmonary Rehabilitation*, **9**, 103–9.

Chapter 6

Leadership, Exercise Class Management and Safety in Cardiac Rehabilitation

Fiona Lough

Chapter outline

The previous chapters have covered the main requirements of exercise prescription, delivery and design. To date there is very little information on the professional competencies and core skills required by exercise leaders to deliver supervised exercise-based CR programmes in the UK. This chapter aims to provide guidelines for UK exercise professionals in CR and addresses leadership roles, class management and safety issues. The focus is on leading phase III CR exercise classes, but much of the chapter is applicable to phase IV classes.

THE UK CONTEXT

Engaging patients in a rehabilitation activity programme and delivering effective exercise require a combination of clinical knowledge, exercise prescription and behavioural management skills. In addition, the exercise leader should have skills of good leadership and organisation of people, exercise locations, equipment and resources.

Exercise-based CR is best provided by a multi-professional team of clinical and exercise specialists able to undertake cardiovascular assessment, individualised exercise prescription, progression and monitoring. This must be in the context of a behavioural approach, in order to meet patients' lifestyle and activity needs.

Exercise Leadership in Cardiac Rehabilitation. An Evidence-Based Approach. Edited by Morag Thow.
Copyright 2006 by John Wiley & Sons Ltd. ISBN 0-470-01971-9

Competencies and core skills

Guidelines on the professional competencies and core skills required to deliver supervised phase III exercise programmes are provided in other countries, for example, the Australian and American Guidelines (Southard, *et al.*, 1994; Goble and Worcester, 1999; ACSM, 2000; American Physical Therapy Association, 2003; AACVPR, 2004). However, there has been limited work in the UK on describing either the role or functions of CR health professionals or their competencies, qualifications and continuing professional development and the education they require. Under the auspices of Skills for Health and the Knowledge Skills Framework (2004) there is increasing acknowledgement of the need for competency-based programmes for health professionals. However, it is generally accepted that all members of the CR team should hold a recognised qualification, i.e. diploma/degree. Most nurses coming into the speciality would ideally have done so via coronary care or similar background. In most countries the minimum requirement to work in the speciality would be attendance at a short course in CR, many of which are delivered by specific interest groups and professional associations, i.e. BACR. Numerous UK academic institutions now offer modular courses appropriate for CR professionals up to Masters level.

A small survey of phase III CR physiotherapists in the West of Scotland (Thow, *et al.*, 2003) defined some aspects of the physiotherapist's professional role. It established that, in addition to cardiac assessment and exercise prescription responsibilities with patients, the physiotherapists had a considerable role in managing, modifying, advising and educating patients with associated non-cardiac physical conditions affecting their exercise programme. Thow, *et al.*'s (2003) study focused only on the phase III exercise aspect by the physiotherapists. There is a need to expand this study and to incorporate the other professionals involved in CR. The Association of Chartered Physiotherapists Interested in Cardiac Rehabilitation (ACPICR, 2005) is currently developing a competency document for physiotherapists, with guidelines for their role and required knowledge, skills and standard of performance.

A UK survey carried out by Bethell, *et al.* (2001) identified nurses and physiotherapists as the two largest professional groups represented in phase III exercise CR (82% and 76% respectively). There are now significant numbers of exercise physiologists, sports scientists and BACR phase IV accredited exercise instructors (BACR, 2002; Turner, 2005, personal communication) involved in delivering phase IV exercise programmes. Given the broad range of exercise professionals working in the multidisciplinary team, definition of individual professional competencies and the complementary roles and responsibilities within the CR team in the UK is required.

EXERCISE LEADERSHIP CHARACTERISTICS

The exercise leader should have the skills to create a safe, positive, welcoming and non-intimidating rehabilitation environment, so that patients and their partners are encouraged to participate in and benefit from lifelong exercise and activity. It is a real challenge to lead an exercise class while dealing with the wide spectrum of clinical, psychological and behavioural reactions that each individual brings to the group.

The challenge for the CR team involves dealing with CR patients and their families who are experiencing, perhaps for the first time, vulnerability in their physical and psychological health. In addition, they may have misconceptions about the safety of exercise. Thus, all CR health professionals require excellent interpersonal and psychological skills in order to engage patients in exercise, developing their trust, confidence and participation. Health professionals in CR need to establish strong, empathic relationships with patients, dealing with many psychological and emotional responses, including fear, depression, aggression, a cavalier approach, over-dependence, denial, obsessive reaction and poor adherence to exercise and other health behaviours. Good interactive leadership, careful handling of group dynamics, in both small and large group settings, and effective class management can create a positive atmosphere of support and camaraderie resulting in a rewarding 'care of the group by the group' ethos. In addition, leading the whole group during the exercise session provides opportunities to promote general socialising, to introduce teaching points, for example, educating patients on key exercise principles, and to encourage group feedback to reinforce learning.

The exercise leader and team need to combine the art and science of exercise prescription and behavioural change to enhance exercise compliance and promote long-term adherence. The ACSM (2000 p. 245) acknowledge this: *unfortunately exercise testing and exercise prescription are often over-emphasised in relation to behavioural components of the programme*. Effective behaviour change, which optimises secondary prevention, involves engaging people in a commitment to an active lifestyle and generalising the exercise habit beyond the rehabilitation session. Some strategies include integrating personal contracts and one-to-one motivational interviewing (see Chapter 8) into the exercise programme. Although there are many factors that contribute to exercise adherence, there is strong evidence that the qualities of the exercise leader can have an enormous influence on cardiac patient participation (Oldridge, 1988).

A CR exercise leader should be:

- professional, credible, confident and enthusiastic;
- a respected advocate and role model for CR;
- a skilled listener, communicator, facilitator and educator;
- a decision maker, with autocratic or democratic style, as required;

- a motivator with persuasive skills who sets realistic and achievable aims;
- tactful, organised, with a planned, systematic approach, directive as appropriate;
- an excellent manager of time, people and documentation;
- empathic and sincere, an optimist with a strong personality;
- in control of situation creates atmosphere and promotes fun
  (Howley and Franks, 1997; Dalgleish and Dollery, 2001).

Many of the leadership characteristics demonstrated in management of the patient groups are also common and equally important to the professional responsibilities and relationship between the exercise leader and the rest of the CR team.

EXERCISE CLASS MANAGEMENT

With a skilled exercise leader and multi-disciplinary team in place to deliver the exercise session, a comprehensive series of guidelines and protocols needs to be agreed for recruiting and managing patients. This will ensure the necessary clinical information and organisation are in place, prior to and during group sessions. Reference can be made to clinical guidelines, professional standards and competencies in American guidelines (ACSM, 2000; AACVPR, 2004).

For the UK context the following are relevant: BACR (1995), CSP (2002), SIGN (2002) and ACPICR (2003). The most recent guideline is the ACPICR (2003) management of phase III exercise, requiring the following protocols:

- referral and recruitment   (ACPICR 2003 Std 1);
- patient consent   (ACPICR 2003 Std 4);
- induction   (ACPICR 2003 Std 5);
- discharge planning   (ACPICR 2003 Std 10);
- health and safety   (ACPICR 2003 Std 11).

Adoption and implementation of these guidelines require a planned, systematic approach to managing the exercise group. It may be helpful to consider the planning and responsibilities to be undertaken by the exercise leader and team in chronological sequence:

- prior to the exercise class;
- at the start of the exercise class;
- during the exercise class;
- at the end of the exercise class;
- after class members have left the session;
- transition to phase IV.

Prior to the exercise class

It is the responsibility of the clinical exercise leader to meet with the team and ensure that they have had an opportunity to:

- Review and approve clinical information for new patients, to ensure there is
  - adequate information to risk-stratify patient and set exercise prescription;
  - consent for exercise from medical staff, with any contraindications agreed and noted;
  - a review of patient's CR goals, convalescence activity to date and level of physical activity prior to cardiac event;
- Review exercise prescription, clinical status, physical activity goals for current patients and set or revise activity plan as appropriate;
- Collate and review the exercise summary sheet for the patient group to
  - summarise key patient clinical information relating to exercise prescription, e.g. risk stratification, medication, symptoms, resting heart rate and blood pressure;
  - group patients, identifying staff-to-patient supervision ratio and responsibilities at session;
- Identify additional staff responsibilities at session for
  - introduction of new recruit;
  - individual patient exercise test assessment;
  - responsibilities for supporting partners present;
  - mentoring and supervising students or visitors to programme;
- Prepare venue (see Health and Safety section, pp. 168–70)
  - check exercise, emergency and first aid equipment;
  - ensure access and exit points clear; floor/room space adequate, tidy and safe;
  - supply drinking water and emergency glucose drinks and supplements;
  - ensure appropriate room ventilation, temperature and lighting; music set-up, as required;
  - provide partner seating and private area for individual consultation.

(Dalgleish and Dollery, 2001).

Start of the exercise class

Once the exercise leader and exercise team have agreed on the exercise status of the group members and the class environment is ready, the group can enter the class. The exercise leader and team are responsible for the following:

- Meet and greet all patients and partners and welcome to group;
- 'Clerk in' and review all patients:
  - pre-exercise heart rate and blood pressure; blood sugar level, if appropriate;

- clinical status and symptom check;
- medication issues and compliance; confirm advice on non-use of GTN spray at class without first advising and discussing with staff;
- check home activity and completion of exercise diary;
- discuss and review progress on CR goals, e.g. lifestyle and risk factor modification;
- ensure footwear and clothing suited to exercise; no recent alcohol or heavy meal prior to exercising; no chewing gum;
- Patient and CR professional jointly agree patient is fit for exercise session;
- Introduction to class:
  - Welcome and introduce all patients, partners and visitors/observers;
  - Remind participants of general house-keeping arrangements, e.g.
    - timing and plan for exercise session; drinking water available
    - safety issues; fire exits and evacuation procedures.
- Advise patients on importance of pacing of effort and using self-monitoring RPE, recognition of symptoms and responsibility to report any concerns to staff;
- Present induction to exercise programme and environment for new patients to session. A 'buddy' system can be used, where a new member is paired with an established CR participant who guides the new person round the exercise class. Alternatively, a member of support staff can work alongside the new person during session to help them integrate;
- Introduce or revise detail and order of stations in circuit (circuit display cards);
- Have member of staff with responsibility for supporting partners present.

During the exercise class

- Staff act as exercise role models, i.e. clothing, posture, attitude, participating in class (Thompson, *et al.*, 2003);
- Staff recognise and respect the cultural, racial, ethnic and socio-economic diversity within group and consequences for delivery of exercise, e.g. respect for personal modesty, caution with body gestures (AACVPR, 2004);
- Ensure good time and people management, keeping control of the class;
- Maintain safe environment, rigorous observation and monitoring of patients;
- Remind participants that they should use RPE and self-monitoring throughout session;
- Use strong voice, lead good demonstration, positioning and cueing for exercise, ensure patients can hear instructions clearly. The music not too loud or distracting; avoid use of jargon and complicated medical terminology in instructions (see Chapter 7);

- Respond to problem/crisis calmly and efficiently, maintaining patient confidence;
- Ensure individualisation of exercise prescription within the context of the group;
- Promote principles of behaviour change during management of the group
  - Commitment . . . to attend session and participate in rehab goal setting;
  - Monitoring . . . undertake individual patient review and rehab diary check;
  - Reinforcement . . . achievements praised/recognised by professional and peers.

(ACSM, 2001; SIGN, 2002)

End of the exercise class

- Providing an inspiring and motivating closure to the class, praising and providing feedback on the session. Promote home exercise discussing how to generalise activity outside of the session; encourage use of a home activity diary;
- Graduating appropriate patients to community Phase IV programmes;
- Preparing patients for discharge to Phase IV;
- Encouraging questions, discussion and social time after cool-down/recovery; dealing with any questions from partners or family present;
- 'Clerking out' and review patients at end of session.

After the exercise class

- Hold team de-brief meeting;
  - review patients' clinical status;
  - discuss and revise exercise prescription and goals, as appropriate;
  - review potential for onward referral to other team members or health professionals;
  - agree follow-up plan for non-attendees;
  - ensure CR resource and referral material and documentation are regularly updated;
  - plan motivational interview at appropriate stage for patients (see Chapter 8)
- Practise local emergency drill;
- Plan and encourage regular team education meetings and continuing professional development;
- Include relapse prevention by developing coping strategies in anticipation of problems. Discuss adherence difficulties, generalise exercise habit to home setting;
- Deliver an exercise consultation prior to finishing phase III (see Chapter 8).

Transition to phase IV

The phase III team should facilitate the transition to phase IV. Some strategies for encouraging a successful transition include:

- The phase IV exercise leader comes to the phase III class, meets the graduates and may lead an exercise session of phase III;
- The phase III leaders take their graduates to see a phase IV exercise class;
- The phase III sessions are held the first few weeks in the hospital and then in the community. The phase III leader can gradually pass the participants to the phase IV leader depending on the participants' readiness for phase IV.

(Armstrong, *et al.*, 2004).

INFORMATION TO PHASE IV

It is important that, with the patient's approval, appropriate information is passed to the phase IV exercise leader:

- patient details
- GP details
- current medical status
- previous cardiac status
- other health problems
- report on phase III participation
- medications.

HEALTH AND SAFETY ISSUES

Patient safety during exercise is paramount. When patients attend the rehabilitation activity session they are under professional instruction and supervision. Consequently, they are the responsibility of the CR team. Exercise should only be undertaken when the following components of care and associated guidelines for clinical practice are in place: supervision by competent staff, appropriately screened patients, individualised exercise prescription, good class management and a safe venue and environment, with first aid and emergency procedures in place. The following points are collated from recommended national clinical guidelines (BACR, 1995; SIGN, 2002; ACPICR, 2003; AACVPR, 2004). These should be integrated into local protocols.

Staffing

1. There should be appropriate skill mix of professional staff, with specialist training in cardiology, exercise prescription and emergency procedures.

2. There should be a minimum of two trained staff present at all exercise sessions, with the ratio of staff to patients dependent on the risk stratification of the patients and the level of supervision required by individuals within the group. The current UK recommended ratio is 1:5, cited in British Association for Cardiac Rehabilitation Guidelines (1995), Scottish Intercollegiate Guidelines (SIGN, 2002) and national guidelines for the Association of Physiotherapists in Cardiac Rehabilitation (ACPICR, 2003).

3. All staff should have basic life support training, be able to access and use an automated defibrillator (AED) and to place an emergency crash call to either the hospital resuscitation team or to a 999 ambulance call, depending on exercise venue.

4. Exercise training for high-risk patients should be held in a hospital or venue with immediate access to full resuscitation services and a member of staff trained in advanced life support.

5. There should be a policy to ensure that all staff update resuscitation and AED training annually and hold regular practice drills for emergency procedures.

Patient screening and management

6. Comprehensive assessment, risk stratification and exercise prescription must initially be undertaken with each patient and reviewed and revised as required.

7. There should be local protocols defining inclusion and exclusion criteria for the exercise group, a medical consent procedure to participate in exercise and clinical guidelines for excluding a patient with the following contraindications from exercise (see also Chapter 2):
   • Unresolved/unstable angina;
   • New or recurrent symptoms of breathlessness, palpitations, dizziness, swelling of ankles or significant lethargy;
   • Resting systolic blood pressure >200 mm/Hg and diastolic >110 mm/Hg;
   • Significant unexplained drop in blood pressure;
   • Tachycardia >100 beats per minute;
   • Fever and acute systemic illness;

8. All patients should have an exercise induction, be closely observed throughout exercise and for 15 minutes after the cool-down is completed.

Venue, equipment and environment

9. Ensure that adequate accident and injury insurance cover is in place to conduct an exercise group if the venue is outside hospital premises.

10. Ensure that access points to the venue are safe and unobstructed, with emergency exits clearly signed and fire evacuation procedures in place.

11. Ensure that toilets and changing facilities have an emergency call system in place.
12. Check that the venue lighting, floor surface and room space are safe and appropriate, allowing adequate space for a free exercise area, safe placement of equipment and patient traffic around the exercise room (Tharrett and Peterson, 1997; AACVPR, 2004). Specifically, there should be floor space for aerobic exercise per patient of 1.8–2.3 m², and 0.6 m² of space per individual using equipment.
13. CR staff should conduct regular checks on all emergency, first aid, exercise, BP and HR monitoring machines and audio-visual aid equipment. CR staff are responsible for equipment maintenance procedures and for reporting any problems and faults.
14. Temperature and ventilation of the exercise room should be within acknowledged guidelines, so as to avoid potential health risks imposed by heat stress or a cold environment (ACSM, 2000). Specifically, temperature should be maintained at 18–23°C (65–72°F), and humidity at 65% (AACVPR, 2004).
15. Drinking water and glucose drinks or supplements should be available at all times.
16. The facility should provide for confidentiality of patients' records and a private area for confidential patient consultation, if required.

First aid and emergency procedures

17. There should be rapid access to an emergency team, either hospital crash team or ambulance, and a telephone available for raising emergency help.
18. There should be locally agreed protocols for managing emergency situations.
19. A written emergency protocol and plan should be clearly displayed in the venue and drawn to people's attention.
20. Appropriate resuscitation equipment, including a defibrillator, should be available and maintained in accordance with local protocols (see equipment section pp. 175–6).
21. There should be locally agreed protocols to manage symptomatic patients (e.g. angina and hypoglycaemia) and accident or emergency situations.

EMERGENCY PROTOCOLS AND MANAGEMENT OF MEDICAL PROBLEMS

All CR staff should be trained to recognise and deal with signs and symptoms of any cardiovascular incident and be competent to take prompt action to handle any complication that may arise during exercise training (Joint Commission on Accreditation of Healthcare Organisations, 2002a; 2002b). It is the responsibility of staff to minimise the risk of incident by ensuring appropriate patient assessment, risk stratification, induction and supervision of the exercise session. Through vigilant observation, monitoring and prompt recognition of signs and symptoms staff may anticipate problems and intervene to limit or manage an impending medical problem.

Medical complications of exercise training

The evidence of the physiological and psychosocial benefits of habitual exercise in people with CHD is substantial (Pate, *et al.*, 1995; USA Department of Health and Human Services, 1996; Jolliffe, *et al.*, 2004; Leon, *et al.*, 2005) (see Chapter 1). It should be acknowledged that the incidence of cardiovascular complications during exercise is greater amongst persons with CHD than in the general population (Haskell, 1978; VanCamp and Peterson, 1986). Given that more patients at increased risk are now offered CR (Richardson, *et al.*, 2000), it is essential to demonstrate that for appropriately assessed and managed cardiac patients exercise training can be relatively safe (Franklin, *et al.*, 1998). A review of the literature questioning whether the overall benefits of regular exercise outweigh the risk of CV incident concludes, 'The overall absolute risk of cardiovascular complication during exercise is low, especially when weighed against the associated health benefits.'

(ACSM, 2000; p. 13)

However, there are sometimes medical complications.

INCIDENCE OF CV COMPLICATIONS DURING CR EXERCISE TRAINING

Early surveys of cardiovascular complications by VanCamp and Peterson (1986) revealed an incidence of one cardiac arrest per 111 996 patient hours of exercise, 1 MI per 293 990 patient hours and 1 fatality per 783 972 patient hours. It should be noted that these data pre-date the use of revascularisation procedures, improved screening and aggressive contemporary treatment of CHD. More recent studies suggest that the incidence of serious adverse events is low, a USA study citing only four major complications over a nine-year period (one non-fatal MI and three cardiac arrests), resulting in a rate of one complication per 67 126 patient hours of exercise (Vongvanich, *et al.*, 1996). Franklin *et al.* (1998) also report an average incidence of one cardiac arrest per 117 000 patient hours, one non-fatal MI per 220 000 patient hours and one death per 750 000 patient hours of participation. These studies confirm the safety of CR exercise programmes as there are very low mortality and infarction rates during structured exercise.

Emergency procedures

SUDDEN CARDIAC ARREST

It is well documented that the chances of survival following a sudden cardiac arrest are minimal (Herlitz, et *al.*, 2003; Ramaswammy and Page, 2003; Valenzuela, 2003). In Europe cardiovascular disease accounts for around 40% of all deaths under the age of 75 years. One third of patients with coronary artery disease die before they reach hospital (Evans, 1998; Resuscitation Council UK, 2000). In most of these deaths the presenting rhythm is ventricular fibrillation (VF) or pulseless ventricular tachycardia, both potentially reversible by defibrillation. In the USA there are 450 000 unexpected cardiac arrests each year, 25% of which occur in public places (Caffrey, *et al.*, 2002).

The 'Chain of Survival' is a well-documented model for effective cardiopulmonary resuscitation for the past decade (Cummins, *et al.*, 1991; Evans, 1998). It is acknowledged as the 'gold standard' of resuscitation practice. It sets out four components required to achieve survival following cardiac arrest: early access to help, early basic life support (BLS), early defibrillation and early advanced life support.

Given that rapid defibrillation is considered the only treatment for VF, all health care professionals, especially those working in the CR setting, should be trained in the use of automated defibrillators (AED). This is now particularly pertinent to the increasing numbers of programmes held in a community setting, where a 999 ambulance would be the first emergency responder. There have also been developments in public access to defibrillation equipment, largely based on a recent study conducted in Chicago airports (Caffrey, *et al.*, 2002). With ambulance response times of 8 to 15 minutes, they identified average percentage of survival without an AED present of only 5 to 10%. However, with an AED available, and administered within five minutes, long-term survival increased to 67%. With each minute of delay before attempted defibrillation, the chance of a successful outcome reduces by 7–10% (American Heart Association, 1998; Evans, 1998).

Emergency plan

CARE OF A PATIENT FOLLOWING COLLAPSE

All staff are trained in basic life support procedures, with at least one member of staff able to use an AED. As discussed on pp. 168–70 in the Health and Safety section, exercise training for high-risk patients should only take place in a venue where there is immediate access to full resuscitation equipment, and where at least one member of staff is trained in advanced life support. When there is a situation in a class and a patient collapses, there should be an agreed and established emergency protocol with designated responsibilities. The following is an example of a plan of action at a phase III exercise class:

- A local plan of action should be established and adopted as the emergency protocol, where specific responsibilities to manage the emergency incident are assigned:
  Role A   lead nurse responsible for immediate care of patient, delegation of activities to other staff and responsibility for using AED;
  Role B   staff member deemed competent in airways management, responsible for maintaining patient's airway in event of a cardiac arrest and assisting lead nurse in BLS procedures;
  Role C   staff member responsible for emergency call and care of other group members.
- Plan of emergency procedures and appropriate telephone numbers should be displayed in exercise area.
- Hospital crash call or ambulance emergency services (as appropriate) should be advised of the exercise session times/venue in case a call is required.
- Documentation should include a record that regular checks of emergency equipment have been conducted.
- Incident and accident forms should be available and completed, as appropriate.

Emergency plan of action

Once a patient has collapsed, the following steps should be taken:

- assessment by the lead nurse, and BLS commenced as appropriate (Role A);
- emergency help called, AED provided; assistance from other staff (Role B);
- other patients reassured, removed from area and appropriate cool-down and monitoring undertaken by other team member (Role C);
- resuscitation procedures continued until arrival of medical/emergency services;
- clinical details of patient and incident given to medical services by lead nurse;
- care of patient's partner, if present; or contact partner to inform about the incident;
- continued management and reassurance of group before discharge home.

Management of medical problems

CARE OF A PATIENT WITH CHEST PAIN

In the event of a patient experiencing chest pain, the immediate aims are to stop the patient exercising, assess and manage the patient's symptoms and obtain medical help if necessary.

A local protocol should be in place, designating responsibility to the lead nurse to seat the patient and manage the situation, while the exercise leader and other/s continue the class if appropriate. The nurse should:

- seat the patient, away from the main exercising group, in a half-sitting position, with head/shoulders and legs supported (if preferred);
- reassure the patient and assess the nature, scale and duration of symptoms;
- if there is no relief of symptoms within two to three minutes of resting, the patient should be encouraged to administer, or be given, as appropriate, a glyceryl trinitrate (GTN) spray up to three times, at five-minute intervals, following the locally agreed chest pain management protocol. The nurse should monitor heart rate, check blood pressure and undertake a 12-lead ECG, if equipment is available;
- if the angina persists after 15 minutes, either an ambulance should be called, if the class is held in a community setting, or hospital medical help should be summoned immediately in order to assess, treat and admit the patient, as appropriate. The patient should be reassured and monitored closely until emergency medical help arrives, with staff ready to follow protocols for cardiac arrest, should the patient deteriorate. The patient's relatives should be advised of the incident and informed of hospital transfer or admission;
- if the angina symptoms resolve completely with the use of GTN spray within 15 minutes, and in the absence of any other symptoms and with satisfactory heart rate and blood pressure measurement, the nurse may decide that the patient is fit to return to the exercise group. Before resuming the conditioning component of the exercise session an appropriate warm-up must be undertaken, with close monitoring of the patient to ensure there is no recurrence of angina. The heart rate and workload at which exercise-related ischaemia occurred should be documented, and future exercise prescription adjusted by the exercise leader accordingly.

CARE OF A PATIENT WITH DIABETES

Given that exercise has an insulin-like effect, exercise-induced hypoglycaemia is the most common problem for exercising diabetics who take exogenous insulin or, to a lesser degree, oral hypoglycaemic agents. Hypoglycaemia can occur either during exercise or up to four to six hours after exercise. Guidelines from *The Health Professional's Guide to Diabetes and Exercise* (Berger, 1995; Gordon, 1995) cited in ACSM (2000) and AACVPR (2004) advised that:

- a diabetic patient's blood glucose level must be under control before beginning an exercise programme;
- patients should not exercise if blood glucose levels are >300 mg/dL;

- an insulin-dependent patient should have a carbohydrate snack of 20–30 g before exercise if blood glucose is <100 mg/dL;
- blood glucose should be measured before, during and after exercise;
- adjustments in carbohydrate dose and /or insulin may be necessary before or after exercise.

It is most important that patients and staff are knowledgeable about the signs and symptoms of a hypoglycaemic attack. Prompt action in response to signs of weakness, faintness, sweating, pallor, confusion or belligerence can avoid a loss of consciousness.

In the event of a hypoglycaemic episode where the patient is still conscious:

- immediately remove the patient from the exercise environment and sit him/her down;
- administer a glucose drink or supplement to rapidly raise blood sugar level;
- if there is a good response, give more food and drink and allow the patient to rest until he/she feels fully recovered;
- encourage close monitoring of blood sugar level throughout the rest of that day;
- discuss the hypoglycaemic episode with a doctor and adjustment to exercise prescription and/or insulin and carbohydrate dosage, as required.

If the patient loses consciousness:

- summon emergency medical help immediately;
- maintain airway and resuscitation if necessary;
- monitor the patient in the recovery position until medical help arrives. (See more in Chapter 4 on diabetes and exercise.)

EQUIPMENT AND CARE

The type of equipment needed for an out-patient CR service will vary considerably, depending on the style and scale of the exercise programme, i.e. use of gym equipment or circuit design, with or without music, and whether educational or relaxation sessions are included in the programme. The exercise leader may wish to have stock items, such as stopwatch, whistle, exercise instruction and demonstration cards, music (or voice microphone, as appropriate) and heart rate monitors for assessing exercise heart rate.

Emergency and first aid equipment are statutory requirements and should include:

- automated external defibrillator (AED);
- airway adjuncts, e.g. pocket mask or self-inflating bag valve mask (oxygen/face mask may be available to assist handbag ventilation procedure);

- blood pressure monitor;
- stethoscope, wipes and sterile gloves;
- first aid equipment, e.g. ice packs and bandages;
- glucose supplements;
- GTN spray (for use in accordance with local protocol).

Selection, purchase and maintenance of equipment

EQUIPMENT SELECTION

Decisions on the type of exercise equipment should take account of the following qualities:

- needs of the CR group;
- calibration requirements;
- space and safety issues including storage;
- user friendliness;
- purchase and maintenance costs;
- warranties, equipment support and servicing.

The venue dimensions, location of entry and emergency exits, associated 'people traffic flow' and siting of electrical outlets (if required) may all determine the amount, type and choice of equipment or circuit design. CR exercise leaders should also consider the necessity and effectiveness of a piece of equipment to fulfil the exercise objective and assess its suitability for the proposed patient group.

SAFETY CONSIDERATIONS

The safety of exercise equipment should be evaluated in terms of its design, ergonomics, biomechanics and electrical circuitry. There should also be a space allocation of 6 sq ft ($0.6 m^2$) for each individual using equipment. Instructions for use and safety should be clearly visible on equipment. Design of seats and supports should accommodate various body types and sizes, with weight restrictions as appropriate. Apparatus must be constructed to maintain joint movement within normal range, and emergency cut-off switches must be easily accessible (e.g. treadmill). With electrical equipment, all cables and plugs must be secured, covered and sited so that patient traffic is not compromised around equipment.

EQUIPMENT MAINTENANCE

A maintenance programme is important in extending the life of equipment, providing regular safety checks and ensuring the validity and calibration of outcome measures.

LOCATION FOR DELIVERING CARDIAC
REHABILITATION PROGRAMME

The goals of CR are to provide the patient and family with the individualised exercise prescription, counselling, education and support they need to resume an independent, active lifestyle. The majority of patients choose to participate in a clinically supervised phase III programme. They then progress into a long-term phase IV CR programme once they are stable and knowledgeable in self-monitoring and CHD risk factor modification.

However, not all patients are able to, or wish to, attend phase III CR sessions. They may choose to exercise at home because they do not wish to participate in a group, or because of problems of accessing the venue, inconvenience of the venue or programme timing, or because of the cost and time to travel to the programme. In order to overcome the absence of direct supervision and associated peer support, some CR services offer regular telephone contact and mail, fax or internet communication to support, monitor and advise patients through a home-based programme.

Although there is good evidence for the advantage of supervised exercise (Wenger, *et al.*, 1995), home programmes have also been shown to be effective in increasing functional capacity and modifying risk factors (DeBusk, *et al.*, 1994; Haskell, *et al.*, 1994; Bell, 1998). A review of well-conducted randomised trials and observational studies supports findings that

> Low to moderate intensity exercise for low to moderate risk patients can be provided as safely and as effectively in the home or community as well as in the hospital setting. Patients at high risk and those undergoing high intensity training should only exercise at venues with full resuscitation facilities and staff trained in advanced life support.
>
> (SIGN, 2002, p.11)

Increasingly, supervised phase III groups, traditionally held in the hospital setting, are held in the community. Phase III can also be structured to be sited in the hospital for the first half, and in the community for the second half of phase III CR (Armstrong, *et al.*, 2004). This design helps to introduce patients early to a community setting, where phase IV will be based, thus exposing them to a less medical environment and using community facilities. In addition, these may be run as outreach programmes by hospital-based CR professionals, to improve access to services for patients and to overcome space and equipment limitations in hospital sites, or they may be staffed by community health professionals. Recommendations from a British Heart Foundation survey of all CR programmes in England and Wales (Fearnside, *et al.*, 1999) encouraged a joint funding approach between hospital and community trusts in order to improve collaboration between and integration of services and to provide a more economical approach.

The challenge for CR professionals is to match the appropriate programme model to suit the individual patients' needs, overcoming any barriers and limitations, facilitating adherence, maximising benefit and delivering a quality, evidence-based service.

SUMMARY

The leadership characteristics and roles of the exercise leader and assistants have been described for the first time focusing on a UK context. Safety in the delivery of the exercise session and in the use of different equipment is the responsibility of the exercise leader. Protocols for care and use of equipment are also required to be developed by the CR team. Should any medical incident occur, this chapter provides a template for actions to be taken.

REFERENCES

American Association of Cardiovascular and Pulmonary Rehabilitation (AACVPR) (2004) *Guidelines for Cardiac Rehabilitation and Secondary Prevention Programmes*, 4th edn, Human Kinetics, Champaign, IL.

American College of Sports Medicine (ACSM) (2000) *ACSM's Guidelines for Exercise Testing and Prescription*, 6th edn, Williams and Wilkins, Baltimore, MD.

American College of Sports Medicine (ACSM) (2001) *ACSM's Resource Manual for Guidelines for Exercise Testing and Prescription*, 4th edn, Williams and Wilkins, Baltimore, MD.

American Heart Association (AMA) (1998) *Operation Heartbeat Implementation Guide*, American Heart Association, Dallas, TX.

American Physical Therapy Association (2003) Minimum eligibility criteria for cardiovascular and pulmonary physical therapy. http://www.apta.org/Education/specialist/ABPTSCert/minimum_eligibility/cert_cardio [accessed 19 Nov 2004].

Armstrong, G., Dunn, M., Bredin, Y., McCuskey, F., Brown, C. (2004) Patients' views on community cardiac rehabilitation. Proceedings of the British Association for Cardiac Rehabilitation Conference.

Association of the Chartered Physiotherapists Interested in Cardiac Rehabilitation (ACPICR) (2003) Standards for the Exercise Component of the Phase III Cardiac Rehabilitation, The Chartered Society of Physiotherapy, London.

Association of the Chartered Physiotherapists Interested in Cardiac Rehabilitation (ACPICR) (2005) *Competencies for the Exercise Component of Phase III Cardiac Rehabilitation*, CSP, London.

Bell, J.M. (1998) A comparison of a multidisciplinary home based cardiac rehabilitation programme with comprehensive conventional rehabilitation in post-myocardial infarction patients, PhD thesis, London University, London.

Berger, M. (1995) *The Health Professional's Guide to Diabetes and Exercise*, American Diabetes Association, Alexandria, VA.

Bethell H.J.N., Turner, S.C., Evans, J.A., Rose, L. (2001) Cardiac rehabilitation in the United Kingdom: How complete is the provision? *Journal of Cardiopulmonary Rehabilitation*, **21**, 111–15.

British Association for Cardiac Rehabilitation (BACR) (1995) *Guidelines for Cardiac Rehabilitation*, Blackwell Science, Oxford.

British Association for Cardiac Rehabilitation (BACR) (2002) *BACR Exercise Instructor Training Module*, 3rd edn, Human Kinetics, Leeds.

Caffrey, S.L., Willoughby, P.J., Pepe, P.E., Becker, L.B. (2002) Public use of automated external defibrillators. *New England Journal of Medicine*, **347**(16), 1242–7.

Chartered Society of Physiotherapy (CSP) (2002) *Physiotherapy Care and Service Standards*, CSP, London.

Cummins, R.O., Ornato, J.P., Theis, W.H. (1991) Improving survival from sudden cardiac arrest: The 'chain of survival' concept, a statement for health professionals from the Advanced Cardiac Life Support Subcommittee and the Emergency Cardiac Care Committee, American Heart Association. *Circulation*, **83**, 1832–47.

Dalgleish, J., Dollery, S. (2001) *The Health and Fitness Handbook* (ed. Frankam, H). Pearson Education Ltd: Harlow: England.

DeBusk, R.F., Miller, N.H., Superko, H.R., Dennis, C.A., Thomas, R.J., Lew, H.T., *et al.* (1994) A case-management system for coronary risk factor modification after acute myocardial infarction. *Annals of Internal Medicine*, **120**, 721–9.

Evans, T. (1998) Cardiac arrests outside hospital. *British Medical Journal*, **316**, 1031–2.

Fearnside, E., Hall, S., Lillie, S., Sutcliffe, J. and Barrett, J. (1999) Current provision of cardiac rehabilitation in England and Wales. *Coronary Health Care*, **3**, 121–7.

Franklin, B.A., Bonzheim, K., Gordon, S., Timmis, G.C. (1998) Safety of medically supervised outpatient cardiac rehabilitation exercise therapy: A 16-year follow-up. *Chest*, **114**, 902–6.

Goble, A.J. and Worcester M.U.C. (1999) *Best Practice Guidelines for Cardiac Rehabilitation and Secondary Prevention*, The Heart Research Centre, Melbourne.

Gordon, N.F. (1995) *The Health Professional's Guide to Diabetes and Exercise*, American Diabetes Association, Alexandria, VA.

Haskell, W.L. (1978) Cardiovascular complications during exercise training of cardiac patients. *Circulation*, **57**, 920–4.

Haskell, W.L., Alderman, E.L., Fair, J.M., Maron, D.J., Mackey, S.F., Superko, H.R., *et al.* (1994) Effects of intensive multiple risk factor reduction on coronary atherosclerosis and clinical events in men and women with coronary artery disease. *Circulation*, **89**, 975–90.

Herlitz, J., Bang, A., Gunnarsson, J., Engdahl, J., Karlson, B.W., Lindquist, J., *et al.* (2003) Factors associated with survival to hospital discharge among patients hospitalised alive after out of hospital cardiac arrest: Change on outcome over 20 years in the community of Gotenborg, Sweden. *Heart*, **89**, 25–30.

Howley, E.T., Franks, B.D. (1997) *Health Fitness Instructor's Handbook*, Human Kinetics, Leeds.

Joint Commission on Accreditation of Healthcare Organisations (2002a) Hospital. http://www.jcaho.org/htba/ambulatory+care/index.htm [accessed 20 Nov 2004].

Joint Commission on Accreditation of Healthcare Organisations (2002b) Ambulatory care. http://www.jcaho.org/htba/ambulatory+care/index.htm [accessed 23 Nov 2004].

Jolliffe, J.A., Rees, K., Taylor, R.S., Thompson, D., Oldridge, N., Ebrahim, S. (2004) Exercise-based rehabilitation for coronary heart disease. Cochrane Database for

Systematic Reviews.1. [online] available from http://www.cochrane.org [accessed 14 Feb 2004].

Leon, A.S., Franklin, B.A., Costa, F., Balady, G.J., Berra, K.A., Stewart, K.J., *et al.* (2005) Cardiac rehabilitation and secondary prevention of coronary heart disease. *Circulation*, **111**, 369–76.

Oldridge, N.B. (1988) Qualities of an exercise leader. In *ACSM's Resource Manual for Guidelines for Graded Exercise Testing and Exercise Prescription* (eds S.N. Blair, P. Painter, R.R. Pate, L.K. Smith, C.B. Taylor), Lea and Fabiger, Philadelphia, PA, pp. 239–43.

Pate, R.R., Pratt, M., Blair, S.N., Haskell, W.L., Macera, C.A., Bouchard, C., *et al.* (1995) Physical activity and health: A recommendation from the Centres for Disease Control and Prevention and the American College of Sports Medicine. *Journal of the American Medical Association*, **273**, 402–7.

Ramaswammy, J.K., Page, R.L. (2003) The automated external defibrillator: Critical link in the chain of survival. *The Annual Review of Medicine*, **54**, 235–43.

Resuscitation Council UK (2000) *CPR Guidance for Clinical Practice Training in Hospitals*, Resuscitation Council, London.

Richardson, L.A., Buckenmeyer, P.J., Bauman, B.D., Rosneck, J.S., Newman, I., Josephson, R.A., *et al.* (2000) Contemporary cardiac rehabilitation: Patient characteristics and temporal trends over the past decade. *Journal of Cardiopulmonary Rehabilitation*, **20**, 57–64.

Scottish Intercollegiate Guidelines Network (2002) *Cardiac Rehabilitation*, no. 57. Edinburgh.

Skills for Health (2004) Coronary heart disease national workforce competence guide: Version 2. http://www.skillsforhealth.org/chd [accessed 12July 2005]

Southard, D.R., Certo, C., Cosmoss, P., Gordon, N.F., Herbert, W.G., Protas, E.J., Ribisl, P., Swails, S. (1994) Core competencies for cardiac rehabilitation professionals. *Journal of Cardiopulmonary Rehabilitation*, **14**, 87–92.

Tharrett, S.J., Peterson, J.A. (1997) *ACSM's Health/Fitness Facility Standards and Guidelines*, Human Kinetics, Champaign, IL.

Thompson, P.D., Buchner, D., Pina, I.L., Balady, G.J., Williams, M.A., Marcus, B.H. (2003). Exercise and physical activity in prevention and treatment of atherosclerotic cardiovascular disease. *Circulation*, **107**, 3109–16.

Thow, M.K., Armstrong, G., Rafferty, D. (2003) A survey to investigate the non-cardiac conditions and the physiotherapy interventions by physiotherapists in phase III Cardiac Rehabilitation exercise programmes. *Physiotherapy*, **89**(4), 233–7.

United States Department of Health and Human Services (1996) *Physical Activity and Health: A report of the Surgeon General.* US Department of Health and Human Services, Centres for Disease Control and Prevention, National Centre for Chronic Disease Prevention and Health Promotion, Atlanta, GA.

Valenzuela, T.D. (2003) Priming the pump – Can delaying defibrillation improve survival after sudden cardiac death? *Journal of the American Medical Assocation*, **289**(11), 1434–6.

VanCamp, S.P., Peterson, R.A. (1986) Cardiovascular complications of outpatient cardiac rehabilitation programmes. *Journal of the American Medical Association*, **256**, 1160–3.

Vongvanich, P., Paul-Labrador, M.J., Merz, C. (1996) Safety of medically supervised exercise in a cardiac rehabilitation centre. *American Journal of Cardiology*, **77**, 1383–5.

Wenger, N.K., Froelicher, E.S., Smith, L.K., Ades, P.A., Berra, K., Blumenthal, J.A., *et al.* (1995) Cardiac Rehabilitation. Guideline No 17. US Department of Health and Human Services, Agency for Health Care Policy and Research and National Heart, Lung and Blood Institute. *AHCPR publication No. 96–0672*, Rockville, MD.

Chapter 7

Teaching Skills for Cardiac Rehabilitation Exercise Classes

Morag K. Thow

Chapter outline

The previous chapters give the exercise leader both information and practical suggestions on risk assessment, exercise prescription, content and construction for a safe, effective and interesting CR exercise class. There is little literature or guidance on the best practice and skills required not only to lead but also to teach cardiovascular group CR exercise classes. This chapter focuses on the skills required for the exercise leader to teach a CR group class. The chapter reviews preparation of the exercise environment and the group. It will then focus on the teaching skills for delivering group exercise.

PRACTICAL TEACHING SKILLS

Numerous skills are required for teaching a group. Nine aspects of teaching are covered in this chapter. The key components of the skills of teaching group exercise are summarised in Figure 7.1.

PREPARATION

Preparing the class environment

The exercise leader is responsible for the environment where the class will be held. The exercise leader should check prior to the class that the environment is free from any hazards and safe to exercise in. As discussed in Chapter 6 the

Exercise Leadership in Cardiac Rehabilitation. An Evidence-Based Approach. Edited by Morag Thow.
Copyright 2006 by John Wiley & Sons Ltd. ISBN 0-470-01971-9

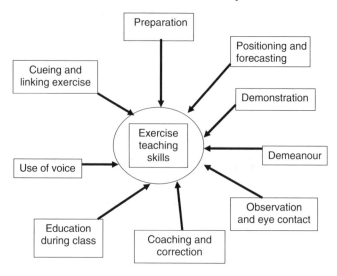

Figure 7.1. Components of exercise teaching.

leader has to check that all emergency equipment and local emergency protocols are in place, with appropriate staff-to-patient ratios. The other support staff members have defined tasks and responsibilities during the class. Any equipment for the class should be prepared, functioning and ready for use. The leader should have prepared the type of class to be delivered, with music and equipment suitable for the class format.

Preparing the class participants

The exercise leader should spend time prior to the class with the exercise team to check participants' current medical status and exercise prescription. Relevant paperwork and data are recorded for each participant on the patient record, including any new symptoms or changes in symptoms since the previous class. Changes in medication or results from tests are also recorded. The class participants' clothing and footwear should be checked prior to the start of the class. The footwear and clothing should be suitable for exercise. New participants should be integrated to the class (see Chapter 6).

POSITIONING AND FORECASTING THE CLASS

The leader should announce that the class is starting. As the leader, you should position and arrange participants to where **you** want them to start. There should be between 1.8 and 2.3 m^2 of space per participant for aerobic activity, and a minimum of $0.6\,m^2$ of space for each individual using exercise equipment. This ensures that there is sufficient space for each CR exerciser. In addition, good spacing will let the exercise leader and assistants best observe participants. If the class is exercising as a group in a free aerobic of activity, it is better to position new people further back. This gives them visual cues from the seasoned class members exercising in front of them. It can also be useful for the exercise leader to stand on a raised platform and check to make certain that the class can see.

Forecasting the class is important, as this is the official start of the class. The forecast is a short section of approximately two to three minutes. The forecast serves many functions:

- sets the atmosphere;
- introduces new members;
- informs on the content of the session and any post-class activities, e.g. talks;
- reminds group of self-monitoring using RPE, breathing perception, etc.;
- reminds group of potential symptoms and actions to be taken.

The following is an example of a class forecast:

Good morning everyone. I am looking forward to our class together. I would like to introduce Frank and Mary who are joining us for their first class. There will be an opportunity to meet them after today's class during tea and coffee. This will be after the talk on healthy eating in the lecture room at 11.30 am.

This morning's class will start with our warm-up to prepare us for our circuit session, followed by our cool-down and stretching. Remember to work in your own comfort zone and Borg exercise level, and that you should be able to talk as you exercise. If at any time you feel any symptoms or become breathless, ease off and report to one of the team. There is water available in this corner. Can you all find a space and make sure you can see me. Can you all see me? Frank and Mary would you like to go to the back beside Fred? We will now start the warm-up.

Once the forecast is complete the exercise leader announces the start of the warm-up.

DEMONSTRATION

Demonstration of the exercise is a vital skill for a successful class (Kennedy and Yoke, 2005). Much of the learning and performance of the group will result from a combination of oral command and visual cues from the leader. Many of the CR group will be over 50 years of age (Bethell, *et al.,* 2001), with age-related physical and motor changes. In addition, hearing is often compromised. Therefore, for many in the group visual cues will dominate as the motor skill learning mode. In order to engage participants whose hearing is compromised, larger, exaggerated gestures should be used to accentuate required exercise manoeuvres. Commands and gestures by the leader should be the same, so as to help the exerciser obtain maximal information for performing the exercises properly. It is important to position yourself to be seen by the class, frequently turning to let the group observe a specific detail of an exercise. For example, turn to face away from the group or side-on in order to let them see how to perform a calf stretch:

> *I am going to turn round. Can you see how my back foot is straight and that there is a space between my feet to help my balance?*

As most motor skill learning results from visual cues, demonstration by the exercise leader must be accurate, as the participants are virtually copying the leader's performance.

Mirror image

When facing the group there is a mirror image: the leader can confuse the group with direction changes of left and right. If you find using left and right difficult, give direction instructions using objects or room features:

> *We are going to move towards the door* or *We are going to take four steps towards the window.*

Similarly, when moving the group forward the leader should move backwards, i.e. same direction as the group. Otherwise, the group will not see the leader:

> *I want you to move forward for three beats and clap on four. Ready, and come forward two, three. . . .* (leader moves back).

DEMEANOUR OF LEADER

The demeanour of the leader is a significant factor in the success of CR, and is regarded by the American College of Sports Medicine (2000) as a major factor in enhancing exercise adherence (Cohen-Mansfield, *et al.*, 2004). The exercise leader must create a happy, pleasant and welcoming atmosphere that is inclusive of the entire group. The leader and other CR professionals should acknowledge people in the class. It can be difficult to remember class members' names. Badges can help the leader recall names and also help class members learn each other's names. This encourages integration into the group, a step which the American College of Sports Medicine (2000) further acknowledges fosters social support, which in turn supports long-term adherence to CR programmes. Furthermore, the leader must appear happy and enthusiastic, with a tone of voice and facial expressions that are positive and upbeat (see more in Chapter 6).

OBSERVATION AND EYE CONTACT

Observation of the class members is a vital skill in exercise leadership. It is the responsibility of all the health professionals involved in the class to observe participants. Observation has many purposes (observation is covered in more detail in Chapter 3, pp. 85–8):

- identifying poor exercise technique;
- identifying subjects over-exercising or exercise abuse;
- recognising safety issues during class, e.g. participants too close to each other;
- assessing performance of group and individuals;
- engaging the group.

It is important that the leader is a vigilant observer, as exercise classes are dynamic; exercise situations and participants change constantly. There should be action taken by observers and class leader in response to the observation.

Eye contact and observing facial expressions of the participants are important for engaging class members, making them feel involved and included. One way to do this is to 'eye scan' during the class. Try not to focus on one person or one group but to scan class members, moving your eye contact round all class members. Eye and facial observation also assists in observation of participants' facial expressions to monitor their exercise effort. Over-exercising or discomfort can often be recognised from participants' facial expressions.

COACHING/CORRECTION

Coaching and correction of the class are the main responsibilities of the exercise leader. Coaching and correction can be directed to specific situations or may be required for an individual. General coaching points are often points that need to be reiterated and take time for motor learning to occur, e.g. for marching:

As you march on the spot, try to land your feet softly on the floor.

This also involves providing ongoing teaching points to cue an exercise so as to ensure that the action or task is performed well. Coaching points can focus on specific body position, performance and technique. Examples of coaching include the following:

- Coaching for 'body listening' exercise perception –
  Remember we should be working at our own level and be able to talk while we exercise.
- Coaching technique –

When you step up on the box, make sure that your whole foot, including your heel, is on the step.

- Coaching the body position and technique for a calf stretch –
  Take a large step back on one foot, toes facing forward.
  Look at your back foot. Check that your back foot is facing forward. Leave a space between your feet to help your balance.

In addition, visualisation can be used to coach activity. Visualisation is where an exercise can be compared to another situation, task or function. For example:

- Coaching using visualisation for a side stretch of the trunk –
  Lean to the side. Slide your hand towards your knee.
  Only move to the side, as if you were between two pieces of glass.
- Coaching using visualisation for a sit-up –
  As you lift your head, keep your chin close to your chest, as if you were holding a small orange between chin and chest.

Many of these coaching elements are ongoing learning points that the exercise leader must repeat often to reinforce the learning and motor skill.

A key point in good teaching is avoiding information overload. When you give correction and teaching commands, allow time for participants to assimilate information. It is therefore important to give clear and short coaching points. Where the exercise performance and technique are being performed either poorly or incorrectly by the class or by an individual, there needs to be correction. Avoid targeting an individual's performance, as this can be embarrassing. Aim the correction and teaching points to the entire group in the first instance. If this is not successful in correcting the exercise, one of the class assistants could give individual coaching. In addition, it may be more appropriate to give an individual a personal coaching period in order to clarify the exercise at the end of the class.

The exercise leader should regularly praise and acknowledge good performance and technique by the group or individuals. For example:

Well done everyone. Our stretching position and balance are improving!
That was a good. We all worked in our training zone.
Well done, Agnes. You have completed two more circuits than you did in your first week.

This helps to reinforce participants' training improvements, learning and motor skills development. Furthermore, successful exercise performance and involvement can enhance participants' perception of self-efficacy (Bandura, 1977) and favourably enhance other future health behaviour change (Ross and Thow, 1997). The exercise leader can help participants recognise such success and see even small improvements as an achievement.

EDUCATING DURING CLASS

Education on the benefits of exercise is a significant role of both the CR exercise leader and team members (SIGN, 2002). The exercise leader should use the principles of adult learning when integrating education during the class (SIGN, 2002):

- relevance   tailored to patients' knowledge, beliefs and circumstances;
- feedback   informed regarding progress with learning or change;
- individualisation   tailored to personal needs;
- facilitation   provided with means to take action and/or reduce barriers;
- reinforcement   rewarded for progress.

These principles should be applied to educating on the benefits of exercise for both cardiovascular and psychosocial improvements. The benefits of exercise are routinely addressed in informal education talks in CR (BACR, 1995). These benefits can further be reinforced and reflected upon during the exercise class. Areas for ongoing education in the class can include warm-up, overload, cool-down, strengthening and self-monitoring skills covered in Chapters 3 and 5. The exercise leader and team members can reinforce and consolidate the benefits and reasons of each section of the class and the content of each. For example:

- reasons for warm-up:
  We are warming up to bring our heart rate slowly up before our more vigorous circuit section. It also helps our muscles and joints to get warmer and we will stretch better.
- benefits of aerobic overload:
  The aerobic section helps us to be able to do more exercise without feeling fatigued.
- reasons for cool down:
  We are cooling down to return our heart rate slowly towards resting.

To review aspects of education during the class the exercise leader can invite the class to answer questions during the class. For example:

Why are we warming up?
Why do we use the Borg scale?

USE OF VOICE

The voice for an exercise leader serves many purposes; it is not, as is often assumed, only for instructing the group. The voice is an instrument that can impart authority, atmosphere and interest to the class, if used well.

Volume

The leader must use enough volume for the group to be heard, often in large spaces with poor acoustics. This can be problematic for CR exercise leaders, who must be aware of the potential to damage their voices (Kennedy and Yoke, 2005). In addition, in a typical week CR exercise leaders can be teaching up to 10 hours (Thow, *et al.*, 2004). There is an extra demand on the exercise leader if he/she is performing the exercise as well as teaching. There is an increased oxygen demand, which could cause the leader to develop laryngitis (Bernardi, *et al.*, 2000). To minimise potential problems, the leader should use good lower torso diaphragmatic breathing. It is important to avoid voice strain by forcing tension on the throat and shoulder muscles. Exercise leaders should also take care not to instruct **all** the time but allow vocal pauses. In large spaces, where acoustics are poor, a voice microphone can be useful to reduce the need for the leader's voice to be used above music and the noise of exercise. A drawback of this method is the cost, insurance and upkeep of equipment. Alternatively, a whistle can be used to attract attention, or, in the case of circuits, to indicate a time change, rather than voice commands. The circuit mode of delivering the aerobic overload period uses the voice in a slightly less demanding way as the exercise leader does not need to communicate to the whole group for the entire session.

Tone and pitch

Tone and pitch of the voice can make it more interesting and can introduce variety and motivational emphasis to the voice. This can work well when emphasising a word or phrase. Using variety also engages the participants, and the leader can use more expression to encourage the group. Varying tone and pitch can be used with emphasis on different types of exercise and can maintain the group's interest and motivation. For example:

For performing a calf stretch, the tone of voice goes down to emphasise pushing the heel into the floor:

> We **push** the heel down into the floor. Can you all **feel** the stretch in the calf muscle?

The exercise leader should also provide the group with information on how different exercises should feel. Variety of tones and pitch can also add to the leader's vocal comfort, avoiding abuse of the vocal cords in sustained use. Furthermore, vocal variation enhances the leader's facial expression, allowing for more flexible movement of the jaw, soft palate, tongue and lips. These are speech organs that shape the leader's outgoing breath into clear, effective speech.

CUEING AND LINKING EXERCISE

In Chapter 5 the different modes of delivery were discussed, with aerobic circuits and free aerobics as key methods in delivery. Often free aerobics will also be used in the warm-up. In free aerobics, where the leader is introducing different combinations and moves with music, the leader is required to link and combine exercises with an element of choreography, i.e. moving in time to the music and facilitating participants to do so. This teaching skill can seem very difficult, as the leader is not only demonstrating and instructing, but also exercising along with the class. As exercise leadership is a motor skill combining many elements, it is advisable to practise moves and combinations of steps prior to taking the class, particularly in the early developmental period of class leadership.

Cueing requires the leader to give the class verbal instruction of the exercise they are about to perform and to fit the exercise to the music. The process of linking exercises requires the leader to move from one exercise to another or to move the group in different directions. To do this there are basic steps, and arm and leg patterns are added to increase exercise intensity (see Chapter 5). When starting to use cueing and linking of free mode of delivery it is best to keep the type of exercise simple and to limit the exercise combinations. Suitable music will have a steady beat with multiple beats of 4, 8, 16, etc. The combinations of exercise can be, for example, basic steps with variety of upper body activity. Basic steps that can be repeated throughout include:

- heel digs for 8 beats
- step back for 8 beats
- knee lifts for 8 beats
- side step for 8 beats.

Each of these combinations needs to be linked together. To manage the transition, the leader can bring the class back to a march between each combination of 8 beats. To start the groups together there are different ways to achieve this, for example:

- count down from four and start on the fourth beat
  Four, three, two and –
- during group marching. The leader demonstrates the move and invites the group to join in
  When you are ready join in.

It is important to remind the group that this type of exercise format is skilful and requires practice. At first they may find it difficult but it will get easier. Furthermore, it is important to point out that the exercises are not dancing (moving aerobically to a rhythm provided by the music). It requires co-ordination and balance, which is good for prevention of falling.

Table 7.1. Tips for developing teaching skills

Tips for developing teaching skills
Watch experienced CR exercise leaders take classes.
Practise with your peers before taking a CR class.
Use a video of yourself taking a CR class to get feedback.
Use a tape recorder to get voice feedback.
Team-teach with an experienced exercise leader.
Take a section of the class and get feedback from experienced leader.
Gradually take more of the class and ask an experienced leader to give you feedback.
Use a mirror to watch your facial expressions and use of mouth.
Attend 'exercise teaching' courses.

Leading free aerobics requires practice and skill. As with any skill, the more leaders can practise the more proficient they will become. A good teacher is not born but develops with practice and experience. There are courses specifically addressing group teaching skills at, for example, the ACPICR and Glasgow Caledonian University. Some tips are given in Table 7.1 to help develop teaching skills.

SUMMARY

Teaching is a critical element for successfully leading CR exercise. Teaching CR well requires awareness and development of many facets in order to develop and maintain proficient exercise leadership skills. An exercise leader may be very knowledgeable on the theoretical aspects of CR, but this is of little use if leaders do not develop and refine their teaching skills to deliver the practical content. The quality of the teacher in health-related exercise is acknowledged as a key element in participants' adherence to and enjoyment of CR.

REFERENCES

American College of Sports Medicine (ACSM) (2000) *ACSM's Guidelines for Exercise Testing and Prescription*, 6th edn, Williams and Wilkins, Baltimore, MD.

Bandura, A. (1977) Towards a unifying theory of behaviour change. *Psychological Review*, **84**, 191–215.

Bernardi, L., Wdowczky-Szulc, J., Valenti, C., Castoldi, S., Passino, C., Spadcini, G., *et al.* (2000) Effects of controlled breathing, mental activity and mental stress with or without verbalization on heart rate variability. *Journal of the American College of Cardiology*, **35**(6), 1462–9.

Bethell, J.N., Turner, S.C., Evans, J.A., Rose, L. (2001) Cardiac rehabilitation in the United Kingdom. How complete is the provision? *Journal of Cardiopulmonary Rehabilitation*, **21**, 101–10.

British Association for Cardiac Rehabilitation (BACR) (1995) *BACR Guidelines for Cardiac Rehabilitation*, Blackwell Science, Oxford.

Cohen-Mansfield, J., Marx, M.S., Biddison, J.R., Guralnik, J.M. (2004) Socio-environmental exercise preferences among older adults. *Preventive Medicine*, **38**, 804–11.

Kennedy, C.A., Yoke, M.M. (2005) *Methods of Group Exercise Instruction*, Human Kinetics, Leeds.

Ross, A.B., Thow, M.K. (1997) Exercise as a catalyst. *Coronary Health Care*, **1**(3), 124–9.

Scottish Intercollegiate Guidelines Network (SIGN) (2002) *Cardiac Rehabilitation*, no. 57. Edinburgh.

Thow, M., Rafferty, D., Armstrong, G. (2004) A UK survey to investigate the physiotherapy involvement and their perceived skills and attributes in the delivery of cardiac rehabilitation. *Physiotherapy*, **90**(2), 97–102.

Chapter 8

Maintaining Physical Activity in Cardiac Rehabilitation

Adrienne Hughes and Nanette Mutrie

Chapter outline

This chapter describes an intervention that has been used to encourage individuals to remain regularly physically active in exercise-based CR in phases III and IV. The principles of this intervention are also appropriate for all phases of CR. This intervention, called the exercise consultation (EC), is based on the Transtheoretical Model of behaviour change and Relapse Prevention Model (pp. 197–205), and uses cognitive and behavioural strategies to increase and maintain physical activity (Loughlan and Mutrie, 1995, 1997).

The strategies used in this EC include: assessing stage of change, decisional balance, overcoming barriers to activity, social support, goal setting, self-monitoring and relapse prevention. It involves a client-centred, one-to-one counselling approach and encourages individuals to develop an activity plan, tailored to their needs, readiness to change and lifestyle. The EC aims to encourage accumulated physical activity accumulating at least 30 minutes of moderate intensity activity on five days per week (Pate, *et al.*, 1995, stage one, as discussed in Chapter 4). In addition, this level of physical activity may be easier for cardiac patients to incorporate into their daily routine and to sustain in the long term. Thus, the exercise consultation encourages individuals to integrate moderate intensity activity into their daily lives. In addition, EC can help maintain involvement in structured exercise in phases III and IV (SIGN, 2002).

ADHERENCE IN CR EXERCISE

It is well documented that exercise-based CR accrues many benefits in patients with established coronary artery disease (US Department for Health and

Exercise Leadership in Cardiac Rehabilitation. An Evidence-Based Approach. Edited by Morag Thow.
Copyright 2006 by John Wiley & Sons Ltd. ISBN 0-470-01971-9

Human Services and Agency for Health Care Policy and Research, 1995; Balady, *et al.*, 2000; SIGN, 2002; Leon, *et al.*, 2005). Achieving these benefits depends on good adherence to cardiac rehabilitation exercise programmes. In addition, sustaining these benefits requires maintenance of physical activity after phase III programme completion. Evidence suggests that improvements in exercise capacity, physical activity and quality of life decline over time following completion of CR exercise programmes (Bock, *et al.*, 1997, Stahle, *et al.*, 1999). Stahle, *et al.* (1999) reported a significant improvement in exercise capacity and physical activity in a group of cardiac patients after three months of supervised exercise training, compared with usual care. However, physical activity levels and exercise capacity had declined in the rehabilitation group 12 months after programme completion (Stahle, *et al.*, 1999). Other studies have found that 50% to 75% of patients do not continue to exercise regularly after completion of formal programmes (Lidell and Fridlund, 1996; Bethell, *et al.*, 1999). Thus, it is important for exercise leaders to implement strategies which encourage adherence to long-term exercise for CR participants to benefit from exercise.

Supervised exercise training in phase III is important in teaching patients to self-monitor their exercise intensity and increase their confidence for exercise. It is unlikely that participation in a supervised exercise programme will facilitate independent exercise after programme completion (SIGN, 2002). This is reflected by the low proportion of patients who continue to engage in regular physical activity after completion of supervised exercise programmes. Therefore, cardiac rehabilitation guidelines recommend that participants in supervised exercise programmes should also incorporate moderate intensity activity into their daily lifestyle in order to encourage regular physical activity in the long term, once the formal programme has ended (Balady, *et al.*, 2000; SIGN, 2002). In addition, the transition from phase III exercise-based cardiac rehabilitation to phase IV can be a challenging time for cardiac patients if they do not receive the support and follow-up from cardiac rehabilitation staff that they received during phases I to III. Instead, patients have to remain physically active independently.

Membership of cardiac support groups that offer group exercise or attendance at phase IV community exercise programmes may help patients to remain active in the long term. However, these exercise opportunities are not available in all areas. Furthermore, some patients may not be able to attend community programmes due to barriers associated with supervised exercise training, including transportation problems, access difficulties (especially in rural areas), inconvenient timing of programmes and work and domestic responsibilities. However, research is limited on effective and practical interventions to encourage individuals to remain active in phase IV.

Behaviour interventions in CR

Exercise consultation was developed in the UK setting. In the US, a similar procedure is termed physical activity counselling. A recent systematic review concluded that physical activity counselling was effective in increasing physical activity and fitness in the general population (Kahn, *et al.*, 2002). Physical activity counselling is also based on the Transtheoretical Model and uses behaviour change strategies similar to those employed in the exercise consultation process. In addition, American CR guidelines recommend that physical activity counselling should be a core component of CR programmes to promote an active lifestyle for patients with CHD (Balady, *et al.*, 2000).

This guideline recommends that physical activity counselling should include an evaluation of the individual's current physical activity level, stage of change for exercise behaviour, self-efficacy, barriers to increasing physical activity and social support in making positive changes. Interventions should include providing support, advice and counselling about physical activity needs, and setting goals to increase physical activity to 30 minutes per day of moderate physical activity on at least five days a week. In addition, patients' daily schedules should be explored in order to suggest how physical activity can be incorporated into their daily routine, e.g. parking further away than usual from entrances, walking up two or more flights of stairs and walking for 15 minutes during lunch breaks. In addition, the use of behaviour change interventions for structured exercise and other health behaviour is recommended in the UK (SIGN, 2002).

BEHAVIOUR CHANGE MODELS

Several behaviour change models have been used to understand exercise behaviour in non-clinical and clinical populations. In addition, these models provide a theoretical framework for developing practical and effective interventions to improve physical activity participation. Although many other models of behaviour change exist, the Transtheoretical Model and Relapse Prevention Model, which are briefly described here, have been extensively studied in exercise settings and provide the basis for many physical activity interventions, including exercise consultation and physical activity counselling (Biddle and Mutrie, 2001).

Transtheoretical Model

The Transtheoretical Model (TTM) was originally developed to understand behaviour change related to smoking cessation (Prochaska and DiClemente, 1983), but has since been applied to exercise behaviour (Prochaska and Marcus, 1994). Interventions based on the TTM have been effective in promoting and maintaining physical activity (Marcus, *et al.*, 1992a; Marcus, *et al.*, 1998a, 1998b; Bock, *et al.*, 2001). The model proposes that individuals attempting to change their physical activity behaviour progress through five stages (Marcus and Simkin, 1994). The stages differ according to an individual's intention and behaviour and have been labelled as follows:

- Precontemplation (inactive and no intention to change);
- Contemplation (inactive, but intending to change in the next six months);
- Preparation (engaging in some activity, but not regularly);
- Action (regularly physically active, but only began in the past six months);
- Maintenance (regularly active for more than six months).

Movement through these stages often occurs in a cyclic pattern because many individuals relapse to an earlier stage when attempting behaviour change.

Three components of the TTM are hypothesised to mediate the behaviour change process: the decisional balance, self-efficacy and the processes of change. Decisional balance involves a comparison of the perceived pros and cons of engaging in behaviour. Studies have demonstrated a significant relationship between exercise adherence and perceived pros and cons of exercise in patients with CHD (Tirrell and Hart, 1980; Robertson and Keller, 1992; Hellman, 1997). A recent meta-analysis (Marshall and Biddle, 2001) found that the decisional balance is related to the stage of exercise behaviour change as depicted in Figure 8.1.

The pros of exercise increase with advancing stage of change, with the largest increase evident from the precontemplation to the contemplation stage. The perceived cons of change decrease across the stages, with the most pronounced decline occurring from precontemplation to contemplation. Therefore, it seems that increasing perception of the pros and decreasing perception of the cons of exercise are important to increase physical activity. Similarly, Hellman (1997) reported a decline in the perceived costs of exercise and an increase in the perceived benefits of exercise, with advancing stage of change in a group of patients who had previously attended in-patient CR.

Self-efficacy was integrated into the TTM from Bandura's Self-Efficacy Theory (Bandura, 1977), and is defined as an individual's confidence in his or her ability to perform a specific behaviour. Self-efficacy is an important determinant of exercise compliance in cardiac rehabilitation settings (Robertson and Keller, 1992; Vidmar and Rubinson, 1994). Findings from the meta-analysis (Marshall and Biddle, 2001) demonstrated a significant relationship between exercise self-efficacy and stage of change, as illustrated in Figure 8.1. The graph shows that confidence to be active increases with each forward movement in stage of change. Individuals in the precontemplation stage demonstrate the lowest self-efficacy, whereas those in maintenance have the highest self-efficacy. Furthermore, the relationship between exercise self-efficacy and stage of change is non-linear, and self-efficacy seems to be

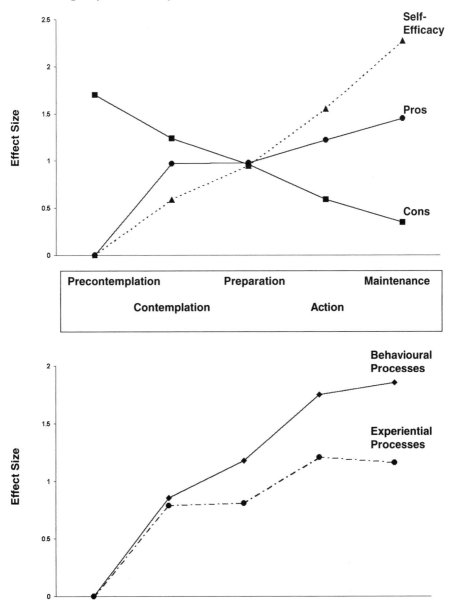

Figure 8.1. Relationship between the stages of change and decisional balance, self-efficacy and processes of change.

(Adapted from Marshall and Biddle, 2001.)

Table 8.1. Processes of Exercise Behaviour Change

Process of Change	Definition (adapted from Marcus, *et al.*, 1992b)
Experiential	
Consciousness raising	Providing information about the benefits of physical activity and discuss the current physical activity recommendations
Dramatic relief	Discussing the risks of inactivity
Environmental reevaluation	Emphasise the social and environmental benefits of physical activity
Self-reevaluation	Review current physical activity status and assess values related to physical activity
Social liberation	Raise awareness of potential opportunities to be active and discuss how acceptable and available they are to the individual
Behavioural	
Counterconditioning	Discussion of how to substitute inactivity for more active options (e.g. taking the stairs instead of the lift)
Helping relationships	Seeking out friends, family and work colleagues who can provide support
Reinforcement management	Rewarding successful attempts at being active
Self-liberation	Making commitments for activity (e.g. goal setting)
Stimulus control	Control of situations that may have a negative impact on physical activity and developing ways to prevent relapse during these situations

especially important when moving from action to maintenance. Similarly, Hellman (1997) reported that exercise self-efficacy is significantly related to stage of exercise behaviour change in CR participants.

The processes of change are strategies and techniques that individuals use when changing their exercise behaviour (Marcus, *et al.*, 1992b). There are ten processes: five experiential and five behavioural. A description of each is provided in Table 8.1.

The meta-analysis (Marshall and Biddle, 2001) found that the frequency of using the processes of change varies across the five stages of change (see Figure 8.1). The use of experiential and behavioural processes increases with advancement through stages, with the largest increase occurring from precontemplation to contemplation and preparation to action. Furthermore, the frequency of using the behavioural processes is more important than that of experiential processes, from the contemplation stage onwards. There is little change in process use from the action to maintenance stages, implying either that maintenance of physical activity does not require further change in experiential and behavioural strategies, or that individuals use additional strategies to those proposed by the processes of change. Similarly, an observational study of patients who had previously attended a cardiac rehabilitation programme found that the experiential and behavioural processes were used more frequently with advancing through the stages of exercise behaviour change (Hellman, 1997).

Changes in the stages and processes of change for exercise behaviour from baseline to six months were measured in a longitudinal study of a group of healthy individuals (Marcus, *et al.*, 1996). At six months, individuals were categorised into four groups: stable sedentary (remained in either precontemplation or contemplation at both assessments), stable active (remained in preparation, action or maintenance at both assessments), adopters (progression from precontemplation, or contemplation to preparation, action or maintenance) and relapsers (regression from preparation, action or maintenance to either contemplation or precontemplation). This study found that behavioural change process use did not change for individuals in the stable active or stable sedentary categories. However, behavioural change process use was significantly greater for individuals who remained active, compared to those who stayed inactive over the study period. Adopters reported a significant increase in the use of experiential and behavioural processes, whereas relapses reported a significant decline in the use of all behavioural processes and one experiential process (dramatic relief). These findings suggest that continued use of behavioural strategies may be important to prevent relapse. Furthermore, a significant decline in dramatic relief among relapses suggests that either belief in the health benefits of physical activity decreases considerably when individuals are no longer physically active, or that inactivity is no longer viewed as an emotional issue.

Application of the TTM in CR setting

Bock, *et al.* (1997) measured the components of the TTM and physical activity in 62 cardiac patients at the beginning and end of a 12-week phase II supervised exercise programme and at three months follow-up. At the beginning of phase II, 43% of participants were in the action and maintenance stages (i.e. accumulating a minimum of 30 minutes of moderate activity on most days per week). At the end of the programme, 96% of participants were in the action and maintenance stages, and self-reported physical activity had significantly increased. Moreover, there were significant increases in exercise self-efficacy and the use of behavioural processes, and a significant reduction in the perceived cons of exercise, with no change in the use of experiential processes or perceived pros of exercise. Three months after programme completion, the proportion of patients in the action and maintenance stages had decreased to 80%, and nearly 50% of participants had reduced their physical activity compared to the end of the phase II programme. Individuals who had regressed at the three-month follow-up had significantly lower scores for self-efficacy and use of behavioural processes, and they had more negative decisional balance scores at the end of the phase II programme, compared to participants who remained physically active at three months. Thus, maintenance of physical activity after completion of a CR exercise programme appears to be associated with changes in self-efficacy, decisional balance and behavioural processes. These findings suggest that interventions based on components of the TTM may promote maintenance of physical activity after CR programme completion.

Application of the TTM in the general population

Interventions based on the TTM are effective in promoting and maintaining physical activity in the general population (Marcus, *et al.*, 1992a; Marcus, *et al.*, 1998a, 1998b; Bock, *et al.*, 2001). Marcus randomised 194 sedentary adults to receive either an individualised, stage-matched intervention or a standard intervention over a six-month period (Marcus, *et al.*, 1998a). The stage-matched intervention involved providing participants with individualised feedback about their physical activity behaviour and stage-matched self-help manuals that were designed to apply the components of the TTM. The intervention involved providing participants with typical self-help health promotion booklets to promote physical activity. At six months, a significantly greater proportion of participants in the stage-matched group were regularly active and had progressed to the action stage, compared to those receiving standard treatment. In addition, the stage-matched group were significantly more active than the standard group at six months. Six months after the intervention period had ended, a greater proportion of participants who had received the stage-matched intervention were regularly active and in action or maintenance stages, compared to subjects who received the standard intervention (Bock, *et al.*, 2001). These findings suggest that an intervention tailored to an individual's stage of exercise behaviour change is more effective than a standard intervention to promote and maintain physical activity in a group of sedentary healthy adults. Table 8.2 describes appropriate strategies for each stage of change.

Table 8.2. Appropriate strategies to use in each stage of exercise behaviour change (Adapted from Biddle and Mutrie, 2001)

Stage of Change	Suggested Strategies
Precontemplation	Raise awareness of benefits of activity and risks of inactivity
Contemplation	Decisional balance (perceived pros and cons of activity)
Preparation	Decisional balance, overcoming barriers to activity, set goals for increasing activity, seeking support
Action	Set goals for regular activity, seeking support, rewards, relapse prevention
Maintenance	Varying activities to prevent boredom, seeking support, rewards, relapse prevention

In summary, the transtheoretical model proposes that by identifying an individual's stage of exercise behaviour change, key components such as the processes of change, exercise self-efficacy and decisional balance can be influenced to encourage stage progression and relapse prevention. For example, maintaining physical activity and preventing relapse may require continued use of behavioural processes and enhancing self-efficacy. A description of how each component of the TTM is addressed during exercise consultation is provided in Table 8.3 (p. 204).

Relapse prevention model

Relapse is a breakdown or setback in a person's attempt to change or modify target behaviour. The relapse prevention model was developed to treat addictive behaviours, such as alcoholism and smoking (Marlatt and Gordon, 1985). The model proposes that relapse may result from an individual's inability to cope with situations that pose a risk of return to the previous behaviour. For example, a former smoker finds himself or herself in a social situation with lots of smokers and is tempted to smoke. Thus, helping the individual to acquire strategies to cope with high-risk situations will both reduce the risk of an initial lapse and prevent any lapse from escalating into a total relapse. Simkin and Gross (1994) assessed coping responses to high-risk situations for exercise relapse (e.g. negative mood, boredom, lack of time) in 29 healthy women who had adopted exercise without formal intervention. The participants' activity levels were measured weekly for 14 weeks. The study found that 66% of participants experienced a lapse (defined as not exercising for one week) and 41% experienced a relapse (defined as not exercising for three or more consecutive weeks) over the 14 monitored weeks. Participants who experienced a relapse reported significantly fewer behavioural and cognitive strategies to cope with high-risk situations, compared to participants who did not relapse. These findings suggest that acquiring effective strategies to cope with high-risk situations may prevent relapse.

Relapse prevention training (Simkin and Gross, 1994) involves teaching individuals that a lapse from exercising (e.g. missing an exercise session) need not lead to a relapse (e.g. missing a week without exercising) and a lapse can be prevented from escalating into a complete relapse (e.g. return to a sedentary lifestyle). The individual is encouraged to identify situations that are likely to cause a lapse. Potential high-risk situations relevant to exercise can include bad weather, an increase in work commitments, change in routine, injury or illness. Individuals are encouraged to develop a plan to cope with these high-risk situations. For example, increased work commitments could be overcome by rescheduling an activity session or engaging in a shorter bout of activity. Such coping is believed to prevent escalation of a lapse into a relapse.

Studies have used relapse prevention strategies to improve exercise adherence in the general population (King and Fredrickson, 1984; Belisle, *et al.*, 1987;

Table 8.3. Description of how each component of the TTM is addressed during exercise consultation

Component of TTM	Exercise Consultation Strategy	Description of Strategy
Decisional balance	Decisional balance table	Perceived pros and cons of being active
Self-efficacy	Exploring activity options and setting goals	Providing realistic opportunities for success and achievement
Experiential Processes		
Consciousness raising	Decisional balance table	Providing information about the benefits of physical activity and discuss the current physical activity recommendations
Dramatic relief	Decisional balance table	Discussing the risks of inactivity
Environmental reevaluation	Decisional balance table	Emphasise the social and environmental benefits of physical activity
Self-reevaluation	Review current physical activity status and assess values related to physical activity	Review current physical activity status and assess values related to physical activity
Social liberation	Exploring suitable activity options	Raise awareness of potential opportunities to be active and discuss how acceptable and available they are to the individual
Behavioural Processes		
Counterconditioning	Exploring suitable activity options	Discussion of how to substitute inactivity for more active options (e.g. taking the stairs instead of the lift)
Helping relationships	Seeking social support	Seeking out friends, family and work colleagues who can provide support
Reinforcement management	Relapse prevention strategies	Rewarding successful attempts at being active
Self-liberation	Goal setting	Making commitments for activity (e.g. goal setting)
Stimulus control	Relapse prevention	Control of situations that may have a negative impact on activity and develop ways to prevent relapse in these situations

King, *et al.*, 1988). Belisle, *et al.* (1987) reported that relapse prevention train-ing increased attendance at a ten-week exercise programme and improved maintenance of exercise for 12 weeks following programme completion (Belisle, *et al.*, 1987). Another study evaluated the effect of relapse prevention techniques to maintain physical activity for six months after completion of a six-month home-based exercise programme (King, *et al.*, 1988). Fifty-one sub-jects were randomised either to receive strategies for improving exercise adherence, including daily self-monitoring of activity and relapse prevention, or to a comparison group who underwent weekly self-monitoring of activity. The intervention group engaged in significantly more exercise sessions over the six-month period, relative to the comparison group. Therefore, daily self-monitoring of activity levels and relapse prevention training is associated with exercise adherence.

Overall, these behaviour change models have been used to understand exer-cise behaviour change in non-clinical and, to a lesser extent, in clinical popu-lations. These theories have identified factors influencing physical activity participation: exercise self-efficacy, perceived pros and cons, use of cognitive and behavioural processes and ability to cope with high-risk situations. In addi-tion, evidence suggests that interventions based on these models are effective in increasing and maintaining physical activity.

CONDUCTING AN EXERCISE CONSULTATION

In 1995, Loughlan and Mutrie published guidelines for health professionals on conducting an exercise consultation (Loughlan and Mutrie, 1995). This inter-vention was originally aimed at sedentary healthy individuals. However, more recently it has been adapted for use with clinical populations, including people with Type II diabetes and CR participants (Hughes, *et al.*, 2003; Kirk, *et al.*, 2004a). This section describes the components involved in delivering the exer-cise consultation to cardiac rehabilitation participants.

Counselling skills

A key element of the intervention is that the consultation is client-centred, which means that individuals should consider their own reasons for being active and should choose their own activity goals. Individuals may be more likely to achieve their goals if they have devised them. In addition, the activ-ity goals should be tailored to the individuals' needs and lifestyle. Good inter-personal skills are essential, which consist of communication (verbal and non-verbal), active listening and expressing empathy. Correct non-verbal communication can be achieved through an open posture (e.g. avoid crossing arms or legs), leaning towards the client, use of appropriate eye contact and a relaxed style to put the participant at ease and to convey interest and attention. Active listening shows the individual that the consultant has listened carefully and understands what he or she has said. This can be demonstrated by 'parroting' (i.e. repeating the key words and phrases that the client used) and paraphrasing (i.e. summarising what the participant has said in your own words). Empathy involves showing individuals that you understand what it is like to be in their world. Empathy can be expressed using examples of other patients who have been in a similar situation to the individual.

As the exercise consultation is a client-centred approach, the consultant should try to avoid preaching, lecturing or providing solutions for the client. The consultant can offer suggestions, such as how to overcome a certain barrier to activity, but this is best achieved by using examples of how other individuals overcame this barrier. Further information on the client-centred approach and the interpersonal skills involved in behaviour change counselling is provided in guidelines on exercise consultation (Loughlan and Mutrie, 1995), and there is also a variety of books on this topic (Rollnick, *et al.*, 1999; Miller and Rollnick, 2002).

COMPONENTS OF AN EXERCISE CONSULTATION

Assessing stage of exercise behaviour change

The consultation should begin by assessing the individual's stage of exercise behaviour change in order to select the most appropriate strategies to use in the consultation. Table 8.4 demonstrates how to assess an individual's stage of change moving from phase III to IV. Those who have recently completed a phase III exercise programme are likely to be either regularly physically active (i.e. in the action or maintenance stage) or doing some activity, but not enough to meet current physical activity guidelines (i.e. preparation stage).

Table 8.4. Assessing stage of exercise behaviour change
(Adapted from Lowther, *et al.*, 1999)

Stage of change	Description
Precontemplation	I am not regularly active and do not intend to be so in the next 6 months.
Contemplation	I am not regularly active but am thinking about starting in the next 6 months.
Preparation	I do some physical activity but not enough to meet the description of regular physical activity given above.
Action	I am regularly active but only began in the last 6 months.
Maintenance	I am regularly active and have been doing so for longer than 6 months.

- Assess stage of change
- Assess current physical activity status (e.g. using a questionnaire or diary)
- Discuss past and present activities to establish likes and dislikes

Decisional Balance Table

Pros	Cons
1. Feel fitter	1. Lack of time
2. Improved well being	2. Don't like walking in bad weather
3. Increased confidence	

Barriers to activity

Barriers to remaining active	Strategies to overcome barriers
1. Less time now returned to work	1. Add some activities into daily routine (e.g. walking part of journey to work)
2. Bad weather (e.g. rain, cold)	2. Do an indoor activity instead

- Review physical activity recommendations
- Explore activity options
- Seek support for activity plan

Goal Setting

1 month	3 month	6 month
1. Brisk walk for 15 mins 3 days/wk	1. Increase brisk walk to 25 mins 3 days/wk	1. Sponsored walk
2. Attend phase IV programme 1 day/wk	2. Attend phase IV programme 1 day/wk	2. Attend phase IV programme 1 day/wk
	3. Swimming once per week for 15 mins	3. Swimming once per week for 25 mins

Preventing relapse

High-risk situations	Coping strategies
1. Busy at work, not enough time to attend class or go swimming	1. Reschedule the swim session or go out walking instead
2. Bad weather, don't want to go out walking	2. Do an indoor activity instead (e.g. swimming or exercise video)

Figure 8.2. Example of an exercise consultation delivered to patients at the end of phase III.

Definition of regular physical activity:

- A minimum of 20 minutes of moderate intensity exercise on three days per week.
  and/or
- Accumulated 30 minutes or more of moderate intensity physical activity on at least five days per week.

The aims of the consultation for individuals in action and maintenance are ensuring that they remain regularly physically active in phase IV and prevent relapse. Figure 8.2 shows an example of an exercise consultation at the transition from phase III to IV.

Individuals in preparation should be encouraged to become regularly physically active. Physical activity recommendations for phase IV participants are
similar to the physical activity guidelines for healthy adults: individuals should
be encouraged to accumulate at least 30 minutes of moderate intensity activity on most days of the week (Pate, *et al.*, 1995) and engage in a minimum of
three 20-minute sessions of moderate to vigorous intensity exercise per week
(ACSM, 1990; 2001).

Assessing current activity levels

Assessing the individual's current physical activity levels can be carried out
using a questionnaire, such as the Stanford Seven-Day Physical Activity Recall
(Blair, *et al.*, 1985), International Physical Activity Questionnaire (IPAQ)
(Craig, *et al.*, 2003) or an activity diary. This assessment provides the exercise
consultant with information on the individuals' actual activities and can be
used to identify possible opportunities for physical activity in their daily
routine (e.g. parking the car further away and walking part of the journey to
work). In addition, daily recording of activities in a diary can help individuals
monitor their progress as they make changes to their exercise behaviour, and
it can provide them with feedback on whether they have achieved their set
goals.

This assessment should be followed by a discussion on the individuals' past
and present activities to discover their likes and dislikes (e.g. if the patient
enjoyed exercising in a group setting, they could attend an exercise class in the
community).

Decisional balance

Participants are asked to complete a decisional balance chart, which involves
comparing the perceived pros and cons of being active. Patients should be
encouraged to identify the benefits gained during the phase III exercise programme. Examples of benefits stated by patients include increased fitness,
improved well being, increased confidence and weight management. The
importance of remaining active in order to maintain these benefits should be
emphasised.

Then individuals should consider additional benefits they would gain by
remaining active in the long term: preventing another heart attack, improving
quality of life, living longer and controlling weight. Patients are also asked to
explore their perceived cons (costs) of being active: examples of perceived
costs of being active experienced by patients include having to make time for
exercise and not liking to walk in bad weather. The aim of the decisional
balance chart is to help individuals realise that the pros of being active outweigh the cons. This is an effective technique for improving exercise adherence (Nigg, *et al.*, 1997).

Overcoming barriers to activity

Patients are also asked to identify possible barriers that may prevent them from remaining active. Some of the individual's perceived cons of activity will be similar to their barriers to remaining active. Many patients return to work after completing phase III exercise training. Thus, lack of time may be a potential barrier to activity in phase IV. This should follow with a discussion on ways to overcome potential barriers to activity. Possible solutions to time constraints include using the stairs, walking part or the entire journey to work or taking a brisk walk at lunchtime.

Social support

Social support is a major determinant of adherence to exercise in CR (Andrew and Oldridge, 1981; Oldridge, *et al.*, 1992). Thus, an important part of the consultation is to encourage individuals to seek support for their activity plan. For example, family or friends could engage in some activity with the individual or praise them for continuing with an active lifestyle. Alternatively, joining a group exercise programme will provide a supportive environment for some individuals. In addition, the involvement of family and partners can help CR participants gain social support to attend phase III programmes.

Exploring activity options

The next part of the consultation involves a discussion with the individual on activities they could do to remain active. The individual's home and work environment should be reviewed in order to see where they could incorporate activity into their daily routine. It may be helpful to have information on physical activity opportunities in the local areas that are suitable for CR patients. For example, the times and locations of indoor shopping centres for indoor walking, or of phase IV community exercise programmes and the times of adult-only swim sessions. Previous discussions on likes and dislikes of activity, current activity status and barriers to physical activity should also be considered. The recommended amounts of physical activity and exercise required to improve and maintain health and fitness, and ways to achieve these recommendations, should also be discussed. As discussed in Chapter 4 the combination of stage one (accumulated activity) and stage two (structured exercise) should be reinforced and discussed.

Goal setting

Setting goals for increasing and maintaining activity in CR is important to help individuals stay motivated. The client should be encouraged to set short-term (one month), intermediate (three month) and long-term (six-month) specific activity goals. The consultant should assist the individual with goal setting to ensure **smarter** goals are set (i.e. specific, **m**easurable, **a**cceptable and **r**ealistic to the individual's lifestyle, **t**ime-phased, **e**njoyable and **r**ecorded). The goals should meet the client's needs and take into account factors discussed during the consultation, such as solutions to barriers, likes and dislikes, and current activity status. Participants should be given a copy of the activity goals to take away with them.

Preventing relapse

Relapse prevention training (Simkin and Gross, 1994) is an important component of the exercise consultation process for patients completing supervised exercise programmes. Relapse prevention training involves teaching individuals that a lapse from exercising (e.g. missing an exercise session) need not lead to a relapse (e.g. missing a week without exercising), and a lapse can be prevented from escalating into a complete relapse (e.g. return to a sedentary lifestyle).

Individuals should be encouraged to identify high-risk situations that may cause a lapse from activity, for example bad weather, increased work commitments or illness. These lapses can accumulate and may lead to a return to a sedentary lifestyle. Developing a plan to cope with these risky situations can reduce the likelihood of a lapse in activity and an overall decline in physical activity, for example, having an alternative indoor activity in bad weather, or rescheduling an activity session or engaging in a shorter bout of activity in order to meet increased work commitments.

REPEAT EXERCISE CONSULTATIONS

Some of the studies evaluating the effectiveness of the exercise consultation have used a repeat exercise consultation at six months. If individuals attend repeat consultations, information recorded during the first exercise consultation should be reviewed. For example, participants should be asked if they achieved the activity goals set during the previous consultation. If clients did not achieve their goals, then the reasons for this should be explored and new goals set. For example, did they encounter any barriers to activity or risky situations that caused a lapse or relapse from activity? Assessing the individuals' current activity levels and comparing them to the first activity assessment can inform individuals if their activity levels have increased, been maintained or declined over the past six months. Individuals who have increased their activity or remained regularly active should be praised for their achievements. However, barriers to activity, problem solving, goal setting and relapse prevention strategies should be discussed with all individuals to ensure they have acquired the necessary skills to help them remain active in the future.

Phone calls can also be used to provide individuals with support for remaining active after an initial exercise consultation. The information recorded during the exercise consultation should be used to guide the phone calls. The phone call may involve discussing any problems the individuals are experiencing in achieving their activity goals, attending community exercise programmes and remaining active.

EFFECT OF EXERCISE CONSULTATION TO INCREASE AND MAINTAIN PHYSICAL ACTIVITY

Several randomised controlled trials have found the exercise consultation to be effective in promoting and maintaining physical activity in non-clinical and clinical populations (Loughlan and Mutrie, 1997; Lowther, *et al.*, 2002; Hughes, *et al.*, 2002, 2003, Kirk, *et al.*, 2004a, 2004b). Lowther, *et al.* (2002) compared the effect of fitness assessment, exercise consultation and standard exercise information on physical activity levels in a group of sedentary healthy individuals. Lowther, *et al.* (2002) found that participants who had received an exercise consultation were significantly more active at 12 months. A recent study of sedentary people with type II diabetes found that the exercise consultation was more effective than standard exercise information in promoting and maintaining physical activity for 12 months (Kirk, *et al.*, 2004b).

Current research provides support for the exercise consultation in CR settings (Hughes, *et al.*, 2002; 2003). A pilot study found that the exercise consultation improved short-term (four weeks) adherence to physical activity after completion of a phase III supervised exercise programme (Hughes, *et al.*, 2003). A recent randomised controlled trial compared the longer-term effect of the exercise consultation with standard exercise information on maintenance of physical activity in 70 cardiac patients who had completed an 11-week phase III supervised exercise programme (Hughes, *et al.*, 2003). Physical activity was assessed using a questionnaire, stage of change for exercise behaviour and accelerometry at baseline (immediately after programme completion), at six and 12 months follow-up. At baseline, both groups were regularly physically active (determined by questionnaire and stage of change), as patients had recently completed an exercise programme. Participation in moderate to vigorous physical activity, measured by questionnaire and accelerometry, was maintained in the experimental group over the 12-month study period. In contrast, self-reported physical activity significantly decreased in the control group from baseline to six and 12 months and total accelerometry counts per week decreased by 8% from baseline to 12 months. Furthermore, a higher proportion of experimental patients was regularly physically active (i.e. in the action and maintenance stages of change) at 12 months, compared to controls. These findings suggest that the exercise consultation successfully maintained physical activity for 12 months after completion of a phase III exercise programme.

Implementing the exercise consultation

Research suggests that the exercise consultation is an effective intervention for maintaining physical activity for 12 months following completion of phase III exercise-based cardiac rehabilitation (Hughes, *et al.*, 2002; Hughes, *et al.*, 2003). Presently, patients completing phase III can attend phase IV maintenance exercise programmes in the community. However, these exercise opportunities are not available in all areas. Furthermore, some patients may not be able to attend structured phase IV programmes due to barriers associated with supervised exercise training, including transportation problems, limited access, work and domestic conflicts. Furthermore, the intervention could be used to facilitate patients' progression from phase III hospital-based exercise programmes to community-based programmes or independent exercise. Thus, the exercise consultation could be routinely provided to cardiac patients on completion of phase III to encourage maintenance of physical activity in phase IV. In addition, exercise consultation has the potential to help patients at all transitions of CR, for example, from phase I to phase II.

Applying exercise consultation to CR

Is it feasible to incorporate the exercise consultation into current CR services? First, the consultations are relatively inexpensive in terms of time, resources and personnel. Exercise consultations last approximately 20 to 30 minutes and the support phone calls five to 10 minutes. In addition, it is possible that patients could record their physical activity habits and the pros and cons of physical activity before attending the consultation, in order to reduce time spent on the consultation. Resources required to conduct the exercise consultation include recording materials (e.g. goals sheet, and guidelines for physical activity) and a quiet room. The exercise consultation could be delivered by a number of health professionals. In the UK, physiotherapists play a central role in the exercise component of cardiac rehabilitation (Thow, *et al.*, 2003).

Physiotherapists have an ideal opportunity to deliver the exercise consultation to patients, as they have good insight, i.e. they are in a position to facilitate the patient's progress from phase I to phase III cardiac rehabilitation and could incorporate exercise consultation into existing programmes. In addition, the transition to the less clinical and supervised phase IV is an ideal opportunity to use exercise consultation. In addition, BACR-trained phase IV exercise staff can use the exercise consultation to provide support to patients who are having difficulty remaining active. In order to be qualified to deliver the exercise consultation, BACR phase IV leaders and exercise leaders require knowledge of the behaviour change theories on which the consultation is based (i.e. Transtheoretical Model and Relapse Prevention Model), and should develop the counselling skills and strategies required to deliver the intervention. This knowledge and skills development can be achieved by appropriate in-service training and/or postgraduate continual professional development (CPD). In addition, individuals need to practise the consultation process.

Training in exercise consultation

Examples of training in exercise consultation have been included in two postgraduate courses for health professionals involved in delivering cardiac rehabilitation services; the first of these is the Rehabilitation in Cardiology at Glasgow Caledonian University aimed at specialist nurses, physiotherapists and other members of the health care team delivering phases I to III CR programmes. The training involves a three-hour lecture on theories of exercise behaviour change, counselling skills and strategies required to deliver the intervention. In the second course, MSc module in Cardiac Rehabilitation for Physiotherapists, there is also a four-hour practical session, where the students have the opportunity to practise the exercise consultation process with cardiac patients.

The exercise consultation has been incorporated into the British Association of Cardiac Rehabilitation (BACR) phase IV training course (Bell, 2000). This course trains exercise instructors to deliver phase IV maintenance exercise programmes in the community for cardiac rehabilitation patients. This course involves a two-hour lecture on theories of exercise behaviour change and the exercise consultation process. In November 2004, the British Association of Sport and Exercise Science (BASES) provided a one-day workshop on physical activity counselling in general and clinical populations, and it is hoped that this workshop will be repeated in the future. Exercise consultation is also taught in several undergraduate and postgraduate Sport and Exercise Science degrees in the UK.

Future research

Many studies have examined the factors influencing uptake of and adherence to supervised CR exercise programmes (Oldridge, *et al.*, 1992; Pell and Morrison, 1998; Dorn, *et al.*, 2001). However, the factors that contribute to maintenance of physical activity during and between phases of CR programmes have not been fully explored. Understanding these factors is an important step in the development of interventions to improve maintenance of physical activity and exercise. Further research in this area is warranted. Similarly, few studies have examined the effect of interventions to encourage long-term maintenance of physical activity following completion of phases II and III CR exercise programmes. Thus, research is needed to test different forms of intervention aimed at improving long-term compliance to physical activity.

Areas that are ripe for further research: Can the exercise consultation maintain physical activity for more than 12 months? Are repeat exercise consultations required? Could the exercise consultation be delivered successfully in a group or by post, telephone or World Wide Web?

The possibility of delivering this intervention to patients in a group setting at the end of phases II and III is a promising area for further study. First, delivering this intervention to groups of patients as an alternative to one-to-one consultations would be more feasible for CR services in terms of time and staff resources. In addition, conducting an exercise consultation in a group setting would provide patients with the opportunity to discuss issues with each other, such as potential barriers to remaining active, problem solving for these barriers and identifying high-risk situations for relapse. Furthermore, group discussion on exercise opportunities in the community, such as phase IV classes, might encourage patients to attend these programmes together. In general, patients routinely receive a discharge interview at the end of phase III that provides cardiac rehabilitation staff with an ideal opportunity to review the patients' goals for remaining active, devised during the group consultations. Studies using physical activity counselling in the general population and other clinical groups have successfully delivered this type of intervention in a group setting (Dunn, *et al.*, 1999; Underwood, *et al.*, 2000).

The exercise consultation may be useful between all phases of CR both to improve adherence to supervised exercise programmes and to encourage patients to participate in physical activity outside of the exercise classes. Patients at the start of phase III are likely to be in the contemplation or preparation stages, and the focus of the consultation should be on encouraging these individuals to increase their physical activity. A pilot study found that web-based and one-to-one exercise consultations were equally effective in increasing physical activity in a group of patients participating in a phase III supervised exercise programme (McKay, *et al.*, 2003).

Other strategies could be included in the exercise consultation to increase its efficacy. Recently, physical activity intervention programmes have found the addition of pedometers to be effective in promoting physical activity (Chan, *et al.*, 2004; Tudor-Locke, *et al.*, 2004). Thus, pedometers, in conjunction with exercise consultation, may be a promising strategy for encouraging participation in physical activity.

SUMMARY

Many benefits are associated with participation in exercise-based CR for patients with established coronary heart disease. Sustaining these benefits requires maintenance of regular long-term physical activity. However, many patients find it difficult to maintain exercise participation and an active lifestyle. The exercise consultation is an effective intervention for maintaining physical activity and could be applied through all phases of CR. In addition, several randomised controlled trials have shown the exercise consultation to be successful in promoting and maintaining physical activity in the general population and for people with type II diabetes. Exercise consultation is based on established theoretical models of behaviour change, and it uses strategies to increase and maintain physical activity. This intervention is practical and could feasibly be incorporated into all phases of CR programmes to encourage patients to remain active. With minimal training, any member of the cardiac rehabilitation team could deliver the exercise consultation. However, in order to be trained to deliver the exercise consultation, exercise leaders need to understand the behaviour change theories on which the consultation is based and the counselling skills and strategies required to deliver the intervention. This would mean that the exercise consultation could be routinely provided to cardiac patients.

REFERENCES

American College of Sports Medicine (ACSM) (1990) The recommended quality and quantity of exercise for developing and maintaining cardiorespiratory and muscular fitness in healthy adults. *Medicine and Science in Sport and Exercise*, **22**, 265–74.

American College of Sports Medicine (ACSM) (2001) *Resource Manual for Guidelines for Exercise Testing and Prescription*, 4th edn, Williams and Wilkins, London.

Andrew, G.M., Oldridge, N.B. (1981) Reasons for dropout from exercise programs in post-coronary patients. *Medicine and Science in Sport and Exercise*, **13**, 164–8.

Balady, G.J., Ades, P.A., Comoss, P., Limacher, M., Pina, I.L., Southard, D. (2000) Core components of cardiac rehabilitation/secondary prevention programs: A statement for healthcare professionals from the American Heart Association and the American Association of Cardiovascular and Pulmonary Rehabilitation. *Circulation*, **102**, 1069–73.

Bandura, A. (1977) Towards a unifying theory of behaviour change. *Psychological Review*, **84**, 191–215.

Belisle, M., Roskies, E., Levesqie, J.M. (1987) Improving adherence to physical activity. *Health Psychology*, **52**, 159–72.

Bell, J.M. (ed) (2000) *BACR Phase IV Training Manual*, 3rd edn, Human Kinetics, Leeds.

Bethell, H.J.N., Turner, S.C., Mullee, M.A. (1999) Cardiac rehabilitation in the community: 11 year follow-up after a randomized controlled trial. *Heart*, **3**, 188.

Biddle, S.J.H., Mutrie, N. (2001) *The Psychology of Physical Activity for Health*, Routledge, London.

Blair, S.N., Haskell, W.L., Ho, P., Paffenbarger, R.S., Vranizan, K.M., Farquhar, J.W. (1985) Assessment of habitual physical activity by a seven day recall in a community survey and controlled experiments. *American Journal of Epidemiology*, **122**, 794–804.

Bock, B.C., Albrecht, A., Traficante, R.M., Clark, M.M., Pinto, B.M., Tilkemeier, P. (1997) Predictors of exercise adherence following participation in a cardiac rehabilitation program. *International Journal of Behavioral Medicine*, **4**, 60–75.

Bock, B.C., Marcus, B.H., Pinto, B.M., Forsyth, L.H. (2001) Maintenance of physical activity following an individualized motivationally tailored intervention. *Annals of Behavioral Medicine*, **23**, 79–87.

Chan, C.B., Ryan, D.A.J., Tudor-Locke, C. (2004) Health benefits of a pedometer-based physical activity intervention in sedentary workers. *Preventive Medicine*, **39**, 1215–22.

Craig, C.L., Marshall, A.L., Sjostrom, M., Bauman, A., Booth, M.L., Ainsworth, B.E. (2003) International physical activity questionnaire: 12 country reliability and validity. *Medicine Science in Sport and Exercise*, **35**, 1381–95.

Dorn, J., Naughton, J., Imamura, D., Trevisan, M. (2001) Correlates of compliance in a randomised exercise trial in myocardial infarction patients. *Medicine and Science in Sport and Exercise*, **33**(7), 1081–9.

Dunn, A.L., Marcus, B., Kampert, J., Garcia, M.E., Kohl, H.W., Blair, S.N. (1999) Comparison of lifestyle and structured interventions to increase physical activity and cardiorespiratory fitness. *Journal of the American Medical Association*, **281**, 327–34.

Hellman, E.A. (1997) Use of the stages of change in exercise adherence model among older adults with a cardiac diagnosis. *Journal of Cardiopulmonary Rehabilitation*, **17**, 145–55.

Hughes, A.R., Kirk, A.F., Mutrie, N., MacIntyre, P.D. (2002) Exercise consultation improves exercise adherence in phase IV cardiac rehabilitation. *Journal of Cardiopulmonary Rehabilitation*, **22**, 421–5.

Hughes, A.R., Mutrie, N., MacIntyre, P.D. (2003) The effect of an exercise consultation on maintenance of physical activity following completion of phase III cardiac rehabilitation. *Heart*, **89**, A23.

Kahn, E.B., Ramsey, L.T., Brownson, R.C., Heath, G.W., Howze, E.H., Powell, K.E. (2002) The effectiveness of interventions to increase physical activity. *American Journal of Preventive Medicine*, **22**, 73–107.

King, A.C., Fredrickson, D.S. (1984) Low-cost strategies for increasing exercise behavior. *Behavior Modification*, **8**, 3–21.

King, A.C., Taylor, C.B., Haskell, W.L., DeBusk, R.F. (1988) Strategies for increasing early adherence to and long-term maintenance of home-based exercise training in healthy middle-aged men and women. *American Journal of Cardiology*, **61**, 628–32.

Kirk, A.F., Mutrie, N., MacIntyre, P.D., Fisher, B.M. (2004a) Promoting and maintaining physical activity in people with Type 2 diabetes. *American Journal of Preventive Medicine*, **27**, 289–96.

Kirk, A.F., Mutrie, N., MacIntyre, P.D., Fisher, B.M. (2004b) Effects of a 12-month physical activity counselling intervention on glycaemic control and on the status of cardiovascular risk factors in people with Type 2 diabetes. *Diabetologia*, **47**, 821–32.

Leon, A.S., Franklin, B.A., Costa, F., Balady, G.J., Berra, K.A., Stewart, K.J., Thompson, P.D., Williams, M.A., Lauer, M.S. (2005) Cardiac rehabilitation and secondary prevention of coronary heart disease. *Circulation*, **111**, 369–76

Lidell, E., Fridlund, B. (1996) Long-term effects of a comprehensive rehabilitation programme after myocardial infarction. *Scandinavian Journal Caring Science*, **10**, 67–74.

Loughlan, C., Mutrie, N. (1995) Conducting an exercise consultation: Guidelines for health professionals. *Journal of the Institute of Health Education*, **33**, 78–82.

Loughlan, C., Mutrie, N. (1997) An evaluation of the effectiveness of three interventions in promoting physical activity in a sedentary population. *Health Education Journal*, **56**, 154–65.

Lowther, M., Mutrie, N., Loughlan, C., McFarlane, C. (1999) Development of a Scottish physical activity questionnaire: A tool for use in physical activity interventions. *British Journal of Sports Medicine*, **33**, 244–9.

Lowther, M., Mutrie, N., Scott, E.M. (2002) Promoting physical activity in a socially and economically deprived community: A 12-month randomised control trial of fitness assessment and exercise consultation. *Journal of Sports Sciences*, **20**, 577–88.

Marcus, B.H., Simkin, L.R. (1994) The transtheoretical model: Applications to exercise behaviour. *Medicine and Science in Sport and Exercise*, **26**, 1400–4.

Marcus, B.H., Simkin, L.R., Rossi, J.S., Pinto, B.M. (1996) Longitudinal shifts in employees' stages and processes of exercise behaviour change. *American Journal of Health Promotion*, **10**, 195–200.

Marcus, B.H., Banspach, S.W., Lefebvre, R.C., Rossi, J.S., Carleton, R.A., Abrams, D.B. (1992a) Using the stages of change model to increase the adoption of physical activity among community participants. *American Journal of Health Promotion*, **6**, 424–9.

Marcus, B.H., Rossi, J.S., Selby V.C., Niaura R.S., Abrams D.B. (1992b) The stages and processes of exercise adoption and maintenance in a worksite sample. *Health Psychology*, **11**, 386–95.

Marcus, B.H., Bock, B.C., Pinto, B.M., Forsyth, L.H., Roberts, M.B., Traficante, R.M. (1998a) Efficacy of an individualized, motivationally-tailored physical activity intervention. *Annals of Behavioral Medicine*, **20**, 174–80.

Marcus, B.H., Emmons, K.M., Simkin-Silverman, L.R., Linnan, L.A., Taylor, E.R., Bock, B.C., *et al.* (1998b) Evaluation of motivationally tailored vs standard self-help physical activity interventions at the workplace. *American Journal of Health Promotion*, **12**, 246–53.

Marlatt, G.A., Gordon, J.R. (1985) *Relapse Prevention: Maintenance strategies in the treatment of addictive behaviors*, Guilford Press, New York.

Marshall, S.J., Biddle, S.J.H. (2001) The transtheoretical model of behavior change: A meta-analysis of applications to physical activity and exercise. *Annals of Behavioral Medicine*, **23**, 229–46.

McKay, K., MacIntyre, P.D., Mutrie, N. (2003) A randomised controlled trial to determine if web-based exercise consultations are as effective as those conducted in person. *Medicine and Science in Sport and Exercise*, **35**, S219.

Miller, W.R., Rollnick, S. (eds) (2002) *Motivational Interviewing: Preparing people for change*, 2nd edn, Guildford Press, London.

Nigg, C.R., Courneya, K.S., Estabrooks, P.A. (1997) Maintaining attendance at a fitness center: An application of the decisional balance sheet. *Behavioral Medicine*, **23**, 130–7.

Oldridge, N.B., Ragowski, B., Gottlieb, M. (1992) Use of outpatient cardiac rehabilitation services: Factors associated with attendance. *Journal of Cardiopulmonary Rehabilitation*, **12**, 25–31.

Pate, R.R., Pratt, M, Blair, S.N., Haskell, W.L., Macera, C.A., Bouchard, C., *et al.* (1995) Physical activity and public health: A recommendation from the Centres for Disease Control and Prevention and the American College of Sports Medicine. *Journal of the American Medical Association*, **273**, 402–7.

Pell, J.P., Morrison, C.E. (1998) Factors associated with low attendance at cardiac rehabilitation. *British Journal of Cardiology*, **5**, 152–5.

Prochaska, J.O., DiClemente, C.C. (1983) Stages and processes of self-change of smoking: Toward an integrative model of change. *Journal of Consulting and Clinical Psychology*, **51**, 390–5.

Prochaska, J.O., Marcus, B.H. (1994) The transtheoretical model: Applications to exercise behaviour. In *Advances in Exercise Adherence* (ed. RK Disman), Human Kinetics Champaign, IL, pp. 161–80.

Robertson, D., Keller, C. (1992) Relationships among health beliefs, self-efficacy, and exercise adherence in patients with coronary artery disease. *Heart and Lung*, **21**, 56–63.

Rollnick, S., Mason, P., Butler, C. (1999) *Health Behaviour Change: A guide for practitioners*, Churchill Livingstone, Edinburgh.

Scottish Intercollegiate Guidelines Network (SIGN) (2002) *Cardiac Rehabilitation*, no. 57. Edinburgh.

Simkin, L.R., Gross, A.M. (1994) Assessment of coping with high-risk situations for exercise relapse among healthy women. *Health Psychology*, **13**, 274–7.

Stahle, A., Mattsson, E., Ryden, L., Unden, A.L., Nordlander, R. (1999) Improved physical fitness and quality of life following training of elderly patients after acute coronary events. *European Heart Journal*, **20**, 1475–84.

Thow, M.K., Armstrong, G., Rafferty, D. (2003) A survey to investigate the non-cardiac conditions and the physiotherapy interventions by Physiotherapists in Phase III Cardiac Rehabilitation exercise programmes. *Physiotherapy*, **89**(4), 233–7.

Tirrell, B.E., Hart, L.K. (1980) The relationship of health beliefs and knowledge to exercise compliance in patients after coronary artery bypass. *Heart and Lung*, **9**, 487–93.

Tudor-Locke, C., Bell, R.C., Myers, A.M., Harris, S.B., Ecclestone, N.A., Lauzon, N. (2004) Controlled outcome evaluation of the First Step Program: A daily physical activity intervention for individuals with type II diabetes. *International Journal of Obesity*, **28**, 113–19.

Underwood, S.J., Barlow, C.E., Chandler, J.L., Kampert, J., Dunn, A.L., Blair, S.N. (2000) Project Prime: 6 month changes in physical activity. *Medicine and Science in Sport and Exercise*, **32**, 97.

US Department for Health and Human Services and Agency for Health Care Policy and Research (1995) *Cardiac Rehabilitation* (Clinical Practice Guideline Number 17), The Agency, Rockville, MD.

Vidmar, P.M., Rubinson, L. (1994) The relationship between self-efficacy and exercise compliance in a cardiac population. *Journal of Cardiopulmonary Rehabilitation*, **14**, 246–54.

Appendix A

GLOSSARY

%HRmax	percentage of maximal heart rate
%HRRmax	percentage of maximal heart rate reserve
%VO$_2$max	percentage of maximal aerobic power
AACVPR	American Association of Cardiovascular and Pulmonary Rehabilitation
ACE	American Council on Exercise
ACE	angiotensen-converting enzyme
ACPICR	Association of the Chartered Physiotherapists Interested in Cardiac Rehabilitation
ACS	acute coronary syndrome
ACSM	American College of Sports Medicine
AED	automated external defibrillator
AHA	American Heart Association
AR	active recovery
BACR	British Association for Cardiac Rehabilitation
BASES	British Association of Sport and Exercise Science
BHF	British Heart Foundation
BLS	basic life support
BMI	body mass index
BP	blood pressure
bpm	beats per minute
CABG	coronary artery bypass graft
CCS	Canadian Cardiovascular Society
CHD	coronary heart disease
CHF	chronic heart failure
CMI	co-morbidity index
COPD	chronic obstructive pulmonary disease
CPD	continual professional development

CR	cardiac rehabilitation
CST	Chester step test
CV	cardiovascular
DBP	diastolic blood pressure
DoH	Department of Health
EC	exercise consultant
EF	ejection fraction
ETT	exercise tolerance testing
FITT	frequency, intensity, time and type of training
FITT (A)	frequency, intensity, time and type of training – adherent
FITT (E)	frequency, intensity, time and type of training – enjoyment
GTN	glyceryl trinitrate
HADS	hospital anxiety and depression scale
HEBS	Health Education Board for Scotland
HF	heart failure
HHP	Have a Heart Paisley
HR	heart rate
HRpeak	peak heart rate
LAD	left anterior descending artery
LV	left ventricular
METs	metabolic equivalents
MI	myocardial infarction
MSE	musculoskeletal endurance
NICE	National Institute for Clinical Excellence
Non-Q	wave that indicates an MI resulting from subtotal occlusion result in less myocardial muscle damage
NYHA	New York Heart Association
OHA	oral hypoglycaemic agents
PC	primary care
PCI	percutaneous coronary interventions
PPL	phonographic performance limited
PTCA	percutaneous transluminal coronary angioplasty
PVD	peripheral vascular disease
RA	rheumatoid arthritis
RE	resistance exercise
RM	repetition maximum
RPE	rating of perceived exertion
RPP	rate pressure product
SBP	systolic blood pressure
SIGN	Scottish Intercollegiate Guidelines Network
SP	secondary prevention
SPECT	single photon emission computed tomography
ST	part of the ECG wave complex that for part of the recording including the P, Q, R, S and T

SWT	shuttle walking test
TTM	Transtheoretical Model
VA	ventricular arrhythmias
VF	ventricular fibrillation
VO_2max	maximal oxygen consumption
VO_2peak	maximal oxygen values attained in presence of a symptom-limited end point

Index

ACE inhibitors 123, 142
active listening 205–6
active living 98
activities of daily living 100, 101, 110
activity plan 100, 101
acute coronary event 9
  during exercise class 41
  see also cardiac arrest, exercise-
    induced; exercise, adverse events
acute coronary syndromes 3
aerobic exercise 50, 86, 111, 137–8
  aerobic circuit interval training 13
aerobic overload 158
aerobic power 56
  maximal (%VO$_2$max) 50
  reserve 50
aerobic/anaerobic metabolic need 50
ageing
  bone loss associated with 110, 121
  cardiovascular function 120
  exercise frequency, intensity and
    duration during 122
  flexibility 121
  heart rate 120
  lean body mass 110, 121
  motor skill 121
  muscle strength 110, 121
  pulmonary function 120
  weight gain associated with 121
ambulatory monitoring 29
American Association of Cardiovascular
  and Pulmonary Rehabilitation,
  guidelines for risk stratification
  36–7, 47
American College of Sports Medicine
  47

anaerobic threshold 71
angina 3, 28, 55, 174
  anginal threshold 4
  exercise-induced 29, 115
  relieved by GTN 28
angiography, as assessment for LV
  function 30
angioplasty 3
anxiety 10, 13, 48, 73, 99, 100, 121
arrhythmia
  arrhythmic potential 30
  exercise-induced 53
  risk of following exercise 155
assessment 10, 207
  before exercise 33–4
  holistic 33
  of exercise history 37
  of physical activities level 37–8

Bandura's Self-Efficacy Theory 198
bed rest, following MI 99
behavioural change 163, 197–205
  readiness for 38
beta blockers 58, 142
  effect on blood pressure 123
  effect on maximal heart rate 53, 105
  and RPE 76–9
  and target heart rate 61–2
body mass index 123–4
Borg rating of perceived exertion scale
  11, 69, 71, 113
box stepping *see* step test
breathing control 112
breathlessness 55, 69, 70
British Association for Cardiac
  Rehabilitation 2, 7, 11

---

calcium channel blockers 123
Canadian Association of Cardiac
    Rehabilitation Guidelines 19, 22–4,
    31
Canadian Cardiovascular Society 23
cardiac arrest, exercise induced 171, 172
cardiac output 56
cardiac rehabilitation 102–3
    content of 6–7
    defined 1–2
    evidence base 7–8
    exercise intensity 48–9
    exercise programme 32
    medical supervision on site 41
    patient groups 3–6
    patient screening 169, 184
    phase I 8, 9–11, 99–101
    phase II 8, 12, 101–2
    phase III 12–13, 66, 104–9, 177, 196
    phase IV 13–14, 39, 66, 119, 196
    staffing levels 40–1, 168–9
cardiac transplantation 4–5
cardiopulmonary resuscitation 172
cardiovascular drift 66, 67
cardiovascular overload 135–55
cardioverter defibrillator, implanted
    5–6
catecholamines, circulating, increase in
    associated with workload 30
Chain of Survival 172
chest pain 29, 173–4
Chester step test 82
chronic heart failure 4
chronic obstructive pulmonary disease
    (COPD)
    effect of music on exercise for 158
    and water-based exercise 118
circuit cards 143–4
circuit interval exercise 106, 107–9
    active recovery 67, 136, 138, 141
    design/layout for 136–7, 139–40;
        advantages and disadvantages of
        formats 144–55
    duration 140–1
    management and control 144
    staff/patient ratio 137
coaching 187–8
Cochrane review 3, 7

co-morbidity 36–7
    co-morbidity index 36
competence, professional 162
cool-down 67, 116–18, 155–6
coronary artery bypass grafting 3
    resumption of exercise following 100
coronary heart disease
    age-related 110, 119–20
    congenital 5
    management 1
    morbidity and mortality 2–3, 7, 20–1,
        119
    primary prevention 21
    secondary prevention 1, 3, 7, 21
coronary perfusion time and
    abnormalities 29
counselling
    psycho-social 13
    skills 205–6
    see also physical activity counselling
CR-10 scale 69–70
critical power 70
cueing 191
cycle ergometry 49, 82, 85

decisional balance 198, 208
deep vein thrombosis, associated with
    bed rest 99
defibrillation 172, 175
depolarisation/repolarisation mechansim,
    effect of exercise on 29
depression 8, 13, 99, 100
diabetes 125–7
    associated with silent ischaemia 29
dose-response principle 48
double pressure product 56
driving, resumption after MI 35, 100
dyspnoea, exercise-induced 4

ECG telemetry 49
Echocardiography 30, 33
education
    in phase I CR 10–11
    in phase III CR 189
ejection fraction
    and heart rate 57
    LV function expressed as 30
emergency equipment 175–6

emergency plan and protocols 170–1, 172, 173
endurance capacity 56
estimated metabolic equivalents *see* metabolic equivalents
European Heart Failure Group 4
exercise
  aerobic 13, 50, 86, 111, 137–8
  adherence to 186, 195–6
  adverse events 21–2, 30–1, 110, 155, 171–5
  benefits 8, 20
  capacity 196
  after cardiac transplantation 5
  community-based 32, 39, 177, 209
  compliance with 163, 198
  demonstration 185–6
  duration 106
  and elderly 6
  exclusion criteria 33
  exercise consultation 195, 197, 205–10; effects of 211–14
  fatigue 74
  frequency, prescribed 99, 104–5
  history 37
  at home 177
  hospital-based 32, 177
  intensity 105
  long-term 211
  mat/floor work, contraindicated 142
  and minority ethnic groups 6
  mobilising 134
  mobility 103
  mode 75–6
  motivation 73
  overload 99, 115–16
  self-monitoring 11
  tolerance testing 26–8, 52, 53, 100
  training 106, 213
  types 106–9
  and women 6
exercise class
  environment 183–4
  equipment 169–70, 175
  forecasting 185
  management 164–8
  positioning 184–5
  repetition 144
  review 165
  skill mix 168–9
  time 144
exercise intensity 48–9, 105
  and heart rate 55–6
  increasing 87–8
  monitoring 86–7
  progression 55–6
exercise leader 163, 186
  characteristics 163–4
  competence and skills 162
  correction 187–8
  demeanour 186
  observation 85, 187
  responsibilities 165–7
  voice 190–1
exertion
  perceived 70
  as trigger of coronary event 52
  see also rating of perceived exertion

fatigue 4, 67
  muscular 67, 69, 79
  volitional 52, 53
first aid 170, 176
FITT principle 48
  FITT (E) and FITT (A) principle 104
flexibility 155–6
Frank-Starling mechanism 57
free aerobic exercise 106, 109, 158, 191
functional capacity 25–6
  and co-morbidity 36
  measurement of 26–8, 82

glyceryl trinitrate (GTN) spray 29, 101, 174, 176
goal setting 209–10

Have a Heart Paisley 38
health and safety 168–70
heart failure, chronic 3
  and exercise 30–1
heart rate 49, 51
  effect of ageing 120
  effect of beta blockers on 58
  ejection fraction 57
  and exercise 49

maximal (%HRmax) 49–50, 51–4; and
        age 51–2; effect of beta-blockers
        on 53
    and myocardial strain 56
    physiological rationale for using
        49–50
    reserve 50
    resting 50
    safe 54–6
    target zones 54
hospital assessment 10
housework, resumption after MI 101
hyperglycaemia 126–7
hypertension 5, 23, 122–3
hypoglycaemia 126, 174–5
hypotension
    age-related 155
    after exercise 17, 155
    orthostatic 115, 123, 125, 142
    postural 123, 125

immobilisation, morbidity associated
    with 99
information overload 188
International Physical Activity
    Questionnaire 208
interval circuit
interval circuit training and exercise
    66–7, 135
    active recovery during 67, 138
    equipment 67
    rationale for 135–6
ischaemia 4, 57
    beneficial effect of exercise on 4
    exercise-induced 53
    ischaemic burden 29, 31
    ischaemic threshold 4
    residual 103

Karvonen heart rate reserve formula 53,
    58

lactate, muscle-produced 50
    lactate threshold 57, 58, 71
lactic acid 56
    and heart rate recovery 67
    and metabolic recovery 67
left ventricular dysfunction 31, 66, 99

left ventricular function 30–1
    and ACE inhibitors 31

Marfan's syndrome 156
metabolic equivalents (METS) 25–6,
    81–5
mobilisation 9, 11, 100
morbidity, psychological 73
muscle
    decline with age 110
    endurance 109–10
    muscular contraction 114–15
    muscular endurance exercise 138
    strength 109–10
music 156–7, 191
    and COPD 158
    effect on perceived exertion 74
MVO₂ *see* oxygen demand/uptake
myocardial infarction
    anterior 99
    incidence 2, 3
    sex-related 3
    and ST-segment elevation 3
myocardial irritability 29
myocardial ischaemia 28–9
myocardial performance, change in
    57–8
myocardial strain, heart rate as indicator
    of 49, 56–7
myocardium contractility 56

National Services Framework for
    Coronary Heart Disease 9
neuropathies peripheral and autonomic,
    associated with diabetes 125
New York Heart Association 23–4
nitrates 123, 142
non-ST-segment elevation syndrome 3

obesity 123–5
occupation *see* return to work
one repetition maximum threshold
    (1RM) 112
osteoarthritis 127–8
osteoporosis 5, 110, 128
overload 115–16
    exercises 104–9
    principle 48, 104

oxygen
  consumption 30
  deficit 30
  demand/uptake (MVO_2) 56–7, 50, 66, 81, 102–5

peak exercise capacity, as predictor of prognosis or death 26
peak heart rate (HRpeak) 52–4, 58, 63–5
percentage maximal aerobic power (%VO_2max) 50
percentage maximum heart rate (%HRmax) 49–50
percutaneous coronary intervention (PCI) 53
percutaneous intervention 3
perfusion abnormalities 29
peripheral vascular disease 127
peripheral vascular resistance 66
physical activity 98–9, 206
  assessment of 208
  barriers to 209
  counselling 197
  definitions 38, 207
  levels, assessment of 37, 207
  maintaining 211–14
  recommendations for 206–7
  self-reporting 38
physiotherapists
pulse oximeter, used during exercise 49
pulse-lowering exercise 116
pulse-raising exercise 102, 134

radial pulse 49
rate pressure product (RPP) 56, 57, 112–13
rating of perceived exertion (RPE) 68–81
  and ambient environment 74–5
  effect of music on 158
  estimation mode 72
  inflation 74
  production mode 72–3
  and psychological status 73
  scale 69, 70
  target 71
  validity and reliability 70–9

and ventilatory/lactate threshold 57
relapse prevention 203, 205, 210
repeat exercise consultation 210–11
resistance training 13, 109–16
  and blood pressure 113
  commencement 111
  contraindications 110–11
  duration 113–14
  equipment 115
  frequency 111
  and heart rate 112
  and high-risk patients 110
  intensity 111–12
  monitoring 112–13
  and women 110
return to work 8, 35, 100, 209
revascularisation 3, 53
rheumatoid arthritis 127–8
risk markers 23
risk stratification 13, 19–20
  components 24–31
  continuous assessment 38
  definition 20
  post-rehabilitation 39
  process 22–4
rowing ergometry 85

Scottish Intercollegiate Guidelines Network guidelines 2, 7, 28, 47
self-efficacy 8, 37, 48, 198–200
self-monitoring 11, 68, 196
sexual activity, resumption after MI 8, 101–2
shuttle walking test 28, 82, 83–4
silent ischaemia 29, 53, 54
  associated with diabetes 126
  see also ischaemia
Skills for Health and the Knowledge of Skills Framework 162
smoking 2, 23
social support 101–2, 209
sodium-potassium balance and myocardial irritability 29
stable angina 4
stage of change model 38
Stanford Seven-Day Physical Activity Recall 208
steady state exercise 106, 107

228 *Exercise Leadership in Cardiac Rehabilitation*

step tests 82
stress testing 28
stretches, stretching 103, 155–6
  during cool-down 117
stroke volume 56, 57, 66
ST-segment
  change 29
  displacement 29, 52
  elevation 3
symptoms, cardiac-related, baseline 34
systolic pressure 56

target heart rate 52, 55, 58, 59–60
  response nuances 66–8
teaching skills 183, 184
training threshold 135
Transtheoretical Model 197–203

treadmill test and exercise 27, 53, 67–8, 72

valsalva manoeuvre 112, 156
valve surgery 5
venous pooling 115, 155
ventilatory threshold 57
ventricular arrhythmia 30
ventricular fibrillation and tachycardia 21, 30, 172
  exercise-induced 30
ventricular filling 57
visualisation 188

walking plan 101
  home walking programme 11
warm-up 102–3, 133–5
water-based exercises 74–5, 117–18, 125